WIVING

WIVING

A Memoir of Loving Then Leaving the Patriarchy

Caitlin Myer

ARCADE PUBLISHING · NEW YORK

First edition

Arcade Publishing books may be purchased in bulk at special discounts for sales promotion, corporate gifts, fund-raising, or educational purposes. Special editions can also be created to specifications. For details, contact the Special Sales Department, Arcade Publishing, 307 West 36th Street, 11th Floor, New York, NY 10018 or arcade@skyhorsepublishing.com.

Arcade Publishing® is a registered trademark of Skyhorse Publishing, Inc.®, a Delaware corporation.

Visit our website at www.arcadepub.com.
Visit the author's website at caitlinmyer.com.

10 9 8 7 6 5 4 3 2 1

Library of Congress Cataloging-in-Publication Data is available on file.

Cover design by Erin Seaward-Hiatt
Cover photo credit: iStockphoto

Print ISBN: 978-1-950691-47-0
Ebook ISBN: 978-1-950691-59-3

Printed in the United States of America

For Marie. Nothing wastes.

A Note about Memory

When I was writing this book, I had dinner with my brother at a cousin's house. We talked about the blueberry summer at my grandparents' farm, comparing what we remembered. That was the summer, I said, when we took the old blue Falcon out of the barn and drove it up and down Myers Road.

Blue Falcon? said my brother. You mean the old Falcon, the green one?

It wasn't green, said my cousin. Was it?

To settle the question, we called the other brothers and my father. Depending on who was remembering, the car was green, or tan, brown, or even red. I was so certain it was blue that, in my memory, we called it The Old Blue Falcon, as though that was its title. But nobody in the family remembered it as blue. None of us could agree on the color at all.

In this book, I've changed many names and a very few identifying details. Some seeming inconsistencies are intentional. For example, *sluff* is a Utah regionalism for skipping school. The spelling is likely a bowdlerization of *slough*, but I can't say for sure. Yael also appears in the text with two different spellings. She is *Jael* in the King James Version of the bible. In other translations, and more commonly, she is *Yael*. I have preferred *Yael* throughout, except when directly quoting the KJV.

Time has always been slippery for me, and in these pages I have occasionally given it a shape for the sake of the story. I don't know, for example, if we drove the Falcon on the sixth day at the farm; what matters is we drove it, and it was marvelous.

I have a decent memory for conversations, and an ex sometimes referred to my "tape recorder," as I was able to play back entire discussions nearly word for word—which proved to be as unhelpful in a relationship as it is useful in a memoir. All the same, my brain is not, in fact, a tape recorder. The dialogue is faithful to my memory, as far as that goes.

While I've checked in with people who were there and verified facts as I was able, my own memory is my primary source, and no matter what my family says, the Falcon will always be blue to me.

Let thy fountain be blessed: and rejoice with the wife of thy youth.

Let her be as the loving hind and pleasant roe; let her breasts satisfy thee at all times; and be thou ravished always with her love.

PROVERBS 5:18–19, *HOLY BIBLE* (KJV)

Behold their pride, and send thy wrath upon their heads: give into mine hand, which am a widow, the power that I have conceived.

JUDITH 9:9, *HOLY BIBLE* (KJV)

WIVING

WIVING

I AM FIFTY YEARS OLD and have just moved to a seaside town in Portugal. I'm reading in a quiet bar when a man asks why a beautiful woman like me is alone.

What he means is, *What is happening between your legs?*

What he means is, *You are breaking the rules of the story, but I can set you straight.*

What he means is, *I can fill that terrible gap between your legs.*

In the story, a woman who is—according to an occult and capricious geometry of features and culture and a man's particular taste—"beautiful" must be attached to a man. To be unattached at my age is a violation of the story. This man wants an explanation. If my answer isn't plausible, if there is no man waiting around the corner or recently dead or banging a college student, I should be grateful that he is offering me a happy ending.

His desire lands on my shoulders like a bird of prey.

What he means is, *I need you to fill the gap in me.*

I like to be alone, I say.

A single no is not enough. I say no to him, and no again. But I have learned to pull the sting of the no, my smile says, *How charming you are, but your desire has nothing to do with me.*

He offers a ride, and is baffled at my refusal, baffled and offers again and again, as though refusal is just part of the dance, as if I could be worn down to a Yes.

Tonight is lucky. This man, on this night, chooses not to force the issue.

Only a few weeks later in the same town, another man will not give so easily. I've been dancing in a Saturday night discotheque with him and his friends. When I turn to leave, he follows me out to the street. My Portuguese is infant-level, but it's clear that he is insisting that I stay. He makes his hands into a heart shape, holds them over his chest.

Não me abandone, he says. This man is thickly muscled with a shaved head and hard face, and he is pleading with me not to abandon him.

Sozinho, I say, one of the first words I learned in Portuguese. *Sozinho. Eu quero sozinho.* I want alone.

He seems to relent. He leans in for the *beijinhos*, the cheek kiss, but as he gets close he grabs my face and forces his tongue into my mouth.

I push him away, step back, then turn and walk, hot and fast. I wind up and down streets and duck into a friend's club, watch from inside to make sure the man hasn't followed.

A friend asks what's going on.

Being a woman is hazardous, I say.

He looks at me for a beat, then nods.

And then I'm free to walk home alone in the dark of the sleeping town. I have believed in freedom for so long, had felt I'd found it, had arrived at freedom over and over again, but tonight I know it is a perpetually receding goal, Xeno's arrow halving the distance forever.

This is the best I have, a lonely walk through a quiet town.

PART 1: WIFE LESSONS

The women's entire education should be planned in relation to men. To please men, to be useful to them, to win their love and respect, to raise them as children, care for them as adults . . . these are women's duties in all ages and these are what they should be taught from childhood.

JEAN-JACQUES ROUSSEAU, FROM *ÉMILE, OR ON EDUCATION* (1762)

EVERY STORY BEGINS WITH THE everyday. Every day the girl crept from her bed of ashes to clean for her stepsisters. Every day the wives of Manasses and Heber served their husbands. Every day the first woman played naked in the garden. You could call her innocent but the word meant nothing then, innocence only comes to life as the mirror image of sin, reversed left to right.

Every day I woke, carried out of dreams on the sound of my husband's sleeping breaths behind me. Every day sunlight striped the dresser and all the day's responsibilities shouldered into my head, jostling for space. Bed to shower to living room while Gabe slept; read the news on my laptop, comics; wrote a few words before work. I kissed my husband awake before leaving the house, a short walk to the bus in soft morning air. Every day, I swear every day I thought, This is how contentment feels.

Nothing new, I said to my mom on the phone. It's weird, there's really no news. This is happiness, isn't it, Mom?

I had escaped the stranglehold of my childhood religion, escaped Utah, escaped a bad relationship. I was married, and the rupture with my parents healed, free of the stories that harassed my youth, loved in the deepening intimacy of couplehood.

So, said Mom, her voice taking on its coy, joking lilt. When will I hear the pitter patter of little feet?

Mom's half-joke. For years before I married Gabe, it was *You know I have to ask about the M word*. But now that I was safely buttoned up in a marriage, the question shifted to babies. Mom was making fun of herself, laughing at the stereotypical Mormon mom question, but there was longing in her voice.

Well. There's a good school here, I said.

This was the every day. The every day that begins every story, before the ash-smeared girl went to the ball. Before Heber's wife Yael lifted a hammer, Manasses's widow Judith a sword. Before the woman in the garden stuffed her mouth with knowledge, a single sin multiplied inside her womb, giving birth to all of humanity.

This is the time before *Until*. Without *Until*, there would be no story.

The Aughts

I AM THIRTY-SIX YEARS OLD, and I'm bleeding. I finished the white pills two days ago, moved on to the green in my pill pack. My period hasn't stopped. I've been on the pill more than fifteen years; in all that time maybe a smear of reddish black the day after white pills, but today the flow is as full as ever. Three days. Four. Now it's weeks and I'm still bleeding.

A little spotting is normal, says my doctor.

This isn't spotting, I say.

She shrugs, writes me a prescription for a different pill. The bleeding draws in, lessens for two days, three, before flooding out with new energy. It was only taking a breath.

My husband and I have been talking about babies. I mean we're picking carefully around land mines. I mean we're talking around talking about it. Gabe said from the beginning he wanted kids with me, but I sensed a shadow behind his certain words. Last month his daughter came to stay with us for just a couple of weeks. She is growing up, twelve years old, coming into her own as a person, sliding down that terrifying slope into adolescence. I love her visits. We took her out to the rocky shore below Sutro Baths. She painted her shoes and mine with rainbows and stars, and we wore our cheerful shoes as we clambered over wet, shining rocks.

My husband was petrified. On edge like I'd never seen him. If his daughter seemed the slightest bit bored, if things didn't go perfectly, I saw his face, the look of a man who had taken the first step into midair off a cliff. One evening,

I dropped a bottle of red nail polish and shattered it on the kitchen floor, painting bright red across our white tiles. Gabe lost it. His face flushed, he yelled and stomped. I got the mop and led him out of the kitchen. I cleaned the tiles while he sat on the couch in full panic mode, gesticulating to himself. My stepdaughter drew her feet up, tucked her knees under her chin, and went quiet.

We are settled and happy in San Francisco, but Gabe's anxiety seems to be ratcheting up. He stays up long after I go to bed, and when he finally joins me I can hear him fidgeting in the dark beside me. He is lying in bed with his eyes open and I know he is eating himself with worry. He worries about money, about failure, about fucking up his daughter, about fucking up with me, about the war in Iraq, about his ex-wife, about work, about his boss; he worries, he frets, he spins himself into knots and he doesn't know how to move forward, how to even begin undoing his knots. I don't know how to help him.

Maybe it is a bad idea to have children with this man, I think. Maybe it will be the final anxiety, the one that will kill him. (Kill us.)

A week or so after my stepdaughter left, I started my period and it didn't stop.

When I was in college, I had a roommate whose mother died of a vaginal hemorrhage. His father had refused to take her to a doctor, although she pleaded with him. Please, she said, please. My roommate showed me her diary, the breakdown of her handwriting as she grew weaker. The last entry was a single word, barely legible:

Gush.

He was only a kid when she died.

I recently switched to the vaginal cup for my periods. More environmentally aware. Healthier. Better. A big plus for me: it holds more blood than a tampon or a pad, and I've always been a heavy bleeder. You're not supposed to be able to overflow these things. I overflow it. When you soak through a pad or a tampon, it starts as a little leak, some spotting, but this is like sloshing water out of a glass. At night I creep on bare feet to the bathroom, spend the night on the toilet, a book on the floor between my feet. My sleep-deprived mind believes the blood will rush all of my organs out, pull me inside out through the gate between my legs.

Work becomes a challenge, but my job is steady while Gabe's is uncertain, so I keep working. I am wearing cup plus pad or tampon plus pad, and still I have to change the whole lot almost every hour. I pass clots. I mean great clumps of meat slip out of my vagina. It feels sloppy, like I can't keep my body in check. Clots as big as a peach pit, or a walnut. This awful creepy sense of one sliding out and I try to clench and keep it inside but I can't. I am losing blood. I've gone greenish white and my concentration slips out of me with all my blood.

Gabe takes me to the hospital one night and they keep me for hours, give me tests. It's morning and I'm still here, have to call in sick to work. They give me a shot that mimics menopause, and for weeks everything irritates me, like sandpaper on an open wound. My husband touches me in a way I don't like and I have to clench my jaw to keep from snapping at him. Still I bleed.

I stop writing, words on a screen can't hold my interest for more than a few minutes. I Google symptoms. Everything tells me I have cancer. I read teen fiction brought over by a member of my writing group. She has teenage daughters, borrows books from them and brings them to me in a paper grocery bag. I tear through the *Twilight* novels and all their overheated teen romance. I'm in bed, layers of towels under my hips, and I have a sudden image of sparkly Edward between my legs, drinking my blood in greedy gulps. Do vampires like menstrual blood? Surely this is addressed in vampire canon. My giggles are shaking the bed. My husband appears in the doorway.

What? he says.

These books, I say, shaking my head. They're just too hilarious.

It was summer when my stepdaughter came to see us. For Thanksgiving we host a dinner. I make everything from scratch, invite friends from other countries, friends with no family in town. It's a good day, my sweetest dreams of married life alive in conversation and warm light and good food and wine. We laugh and eat and someone breaks a glass and we say, Now it's a party. I forget the gravy and serve the pie before it is set up and blueberries gush dark and hot over everyone's plates.

The next night I get up from the couch and the floor seems to breathe me off balance. Gabe puts me in the car and takes me to the hospital. I am dangerously anemic, get bundled into a room for an emergency transfusion. Gabe holds my hand and jokes with me and the nurses, he keeps all of us laughing. They hook me up and blood pumps cold into me, cold moves in through my veins and chills my body down to corpse temperature, the thin hospital blanket an insult. A transfusion takes a long time. They don't show that part in movies. It takes hours, all night. Gabe goes home to feed the cats and comes back with a story about the car battery. He left the headlights on and had to call Triple A and wait for them to show up and there's no cell service in the hospital so he couldn't reach me and he's sorry he was gone so long and I just hold his hand, glad he's there.

After that first hospital visit, I am shunted from doctor to specialist, through rounds of testing and imaging; I live in waiting rooms, exam rooms, and darkened sonogram rooms, screens glowing in the faces of technicians. One of the several doctors I see says:

So young!

This is after I describe to her the months of hemorrhaging, the days I can't leave the toilet, clots now the size of golf balls that pass from my body.

So young! As though this sort of Grand Guignol is to be expected at some point in a woman's life. But only when she is older, when—the implication is—it doesn't matter.

Time moves and shifts under me. Is it days, a week, weeks later? Gabe and I are sitting in the office of another doctor. She tells us we could try an IUD. It may work. If it does work, she won't be able to tell us why it works, in the same way she can't tell me why I'm bleeding. It is only absurdly recently that women have been included in health studies. For a long time researchers proceeded on the assumption that women were just penisless men with breasts and a uterus. Women's bodies remain comparatively mysterious to medical science. My particular body, this blood, this hemorrhage, this gush, is a mystery, but it's just one of thousands of other mysteries. There's some catching up to do.

The doctor says the IUD has a 30 percent chance of working.

If it doesn't work? I say.

If it doesn't work, we'll have to do a hysterectomy, says the doctor. But we will have to wait six months.

I don't ask why six months. I am playing this out in my head. A 70 percent chance that I will have to live with this bleeding for another six months.

The alternative: hysterectomy.

She leaves the office so we can talk. Gabe's face shows panic. Or is the panic mine? Six more months of bleeding. Six months of teen fiction and Gabe's nonexistent cooking skills.

I can't miss six months of work. I've already missed far too much. They've allowed me this time off, they keep paying me, but it is a small company. They can't afford to pay me for six more months. We need my income. Gabe's is not stable.

I blame my husband. I look in his face and divine what he wants me, desperately, to say.

I say it, thinking I can save him, save us.

I blame myself, too. If I was a stronger person, a better person, I would have said, We'll try anything. One must make sacrifices for a child. Children teach you selflessness. I could have started in that moment.

The doctor comes back, and I say, Hysterectomy.

The surgery is scheduled for January; I need to build up my blood enough before they cut into me, another month of iron pills and red meat and spinach. I join a website called HysterSisters. Hate the cuteness of the name, the sticky pink background of the site, the chummy, clubby look-on-the-bright-sideism. But there are women on the site who bled even longer and harder than I did, women who were unable to leave the toilet for weeks. Maybe I didn't try hard enough. But the decision is made.

Niece of Pride! I say, answering the phone. It is January 13, 2005. Friday the thirteenth.

I say it gently. Once upon a time I called her Niece of Shame, a joking reference to a book I'd read. She had rebelled against the church we were both raised in, rebelled against her Utah world. But she's still in Utah, vulnerable in her outsider status, brave in her decision to stay. The joke turned flat. So she became Niece of Pride.

Grandma's dying, she says.

My brain takes a few seconds to align itself. Grandma to my niece, as in Mom. Mom is dying. Her kidneys are failing. She isn't expected to live out the day.

My husband sees something in my face and he stops whatever he was doing.

This is real, I think. This is a real thing.

I know my niece has a lot of other people to call. I thank her. I am strangely formal, I thank her for being the person to tell me. The thing to do in a time like this is cry, but the news hasn't settled inside me yet.

My surgery is in one week. I call the doctor and she says, Of course you have to go.

She gives me a prescription for five different contraceptives. I am to take them all at once in hopes it will slow the bleeding enough for me to travel. We have breakfast at Howard's Café with our friends, because we'd already planned our breakfast date, because you have to eat, because I haven't had the energy to cook in weeks. We walk half a block from the café to the last travel agency in town, book a flight to Salt Lake City for that day. We pack and drive to the airport and I make a sad almost-joke, a Mom-like half-joke to the man at airport security. When he asks why we are flying with a ticket we bought that day, I tell him my mom is dying.

Why are you smiling, he says.

Because I'm from Utah, I say. That's what we do.

We are waiting to board when my phone rings.

Mom is dead.

All my siblings are in the living room, Dad with us. My brothers with their legs stretched long in front of them. It's dark outside the big windows and we are in our fishbowl, and it feels good to be together.

A brother suggests we go to a movie.

Oh, says Dad. You go on without me, I can't leave—

Oh, he says again. He puts his hands on his head. I was going to say I can't leave your mother, but I'm free now. I'm free.

His blue eyes are open wide and tears are falling out of them and his hands are on his bald head. He can go anywhere he wants now. He laughs once, a short, hard laugh. We all feel it, the terrible beauty of his new freedom.

Mom was thirty-six when she had me; I am thirty-six now. This is too tidy. It wouldn't fly in a novel, too weighted with too much meaning. I buzzed my hair short when I first got sick, didn't want to worry about my hair. I started going gray years before and had dyed it ever since. But now I am letting the gray grow in. In a week I will have moved into that sexless territory, a crone at thirty-six. If I believed in God I would call this divine judgment for my sins. I do not believe in God but it seems I still believe in sin. I believe I pulled this onto my own head, and now Mom is gone and I can't talk to her, can't know what she would say. We were just getting to the good part, we were just learning how to say what was in our hearts.

Or maybe I only tell myself that now because she's gone.

Mom has the best laugh. Had. Her laugh pulled you into a small room, just you and her, an exclusive place, warm and full of light, the two of you the only ones in on the joke, her sad half-joke, her way of saying what she meant without taking responsibility for it.

Years later, Dad will say he told her about the hysterectomy. I kick the walls of my memory. Did I talk to her about this? Did I tell her I worried I was doing something wrong? It was a choice but it didn't feel like a choice. Did I ask Mom for absolution, as though it was in her power to forgive my sins, as though she was the one, the only one who could absolve me of the sin of wanting to live? I know she said she loved me. But maybe I heard it only through Dad's voice.

Dad's tired dad voice: Your mother isn't feeling up to talking just now. She loves you, sweetie.

And here we are, in our lighted glass room on a dark January night, my brothers with their long legs. We are making Myer jokes, bad puns, Dad remembers she is gone and then remembers again, he puts his hands on his head and opens his mouth wide with grief.

I love her so much, he says.

Loved her, he says. He shakes his head.

Love her, he says.

Oh, Marie, he says, tears running down his face.

1974

MOM AND DAD'S LOVE STORY was the size of myth, told over and over when I was a kid, as familiar and comforting as Mary and Joseph and the baby in the manger.

I thought I'd have to settle for a righteous cowboy, says Mom.

I'm six years old. We're in the bedroom. Mom's propped up on the pillows, Dad next to her, his pale feet bare. I'm repelled by Dad's bare feet. There's something unmasculine about them. They are entirely too soft, too white, too heavily veined. Mom's feet are hard and rough as a sanding block, though she hardly ever goes outside. She says it's from a lifetime of going barefoot, and to me this is the way feet should be. Dad's are abominations.

We kids are sprawled around the bed.

And then I left the ranch, she says.

She went to college at Brigham Young University, met Dad. He was the art editor for the student literary magazine, she the literary editor. For their first date, he took her out to the ballet in Salt Lake City. The ballet! Head over heels. In her journals she called him Pierre, a sophisticate from New York, although to be accurate he spent his childhood in Ozone Park, Queens, then moved to New Jersey.

Well, he was head over heels. Mom took a little longer. They met several times before it took. They put it all together later. The first time, Mom was with her watercolor class out at the Provo River. Dad swimming the river

13

with friends. He saw the cute chick at her easel and sauntered up, offered some suggestions on her watercolor.

I was kibitzing, says Dad.

I thought you were some snotty high school kid, says Mom. Trying to tell me how to paint.

Mom is stroking the top of Dad's bald head. He looks about ready to purr, eyes half-closed. They tell us about French class. This was one of those crowded classes where you never learn everyone's name. Dad did some sketches of a girl in a ponytail as she gave a report. He still has those. Mom in her glasses and tight sweater. He's sketched the lenses blank, you can't see her eyes. She looks cool and distant.

French was right after my sculpture class, says Dad.

He showed up in dirty jeans with clay on his shoes. I paid him no attention, says Mom.

Except Fridays, when I had ROTC, says Dad. He pronounces it *ROT-see*.

Oh, you looked sharp in that uniform! says Mom.

We have a yearbook picture of the literary magazine staff, the first time they met for real. In the picture, they look young and bright. Dad gave Mom a ride home that night, and that's when he asked her out to the ballet.

Even with the ballet, once Dad got around to proposing, he had competition. Churchy.

Churchy was the better dancer, says Mom. But Peter, she says. Well, some things are more important than dancing.

She raises one eyebrow and cuts her eyes at him. Not that I knew anything about that, she says.

Oh no, says Dad. Certainly not. A-HEM.

Can't you just picture us, says Mom. We got married in the St. George Temple, reception in Mother and Daddy's back yard. We finally got free of all the guests and we're in the car.

We're going out to the ranch for our wedding night, says Dad.

And the car radio's playing, says Mom.

"Unchained Melody" comes on, says Dad.

Think about it, says Mom. Two *starving* virgins . . .

Driving as fast as we can in the dark . . .
And this song. This song! Too much.
Of course it's our song.
I mean, you want to talk sexy, says Mom.

The church tells us a wife must be a homemaker, nurturer, spiritual example for her children, ever cheerful for her husband. Mom rarely makes it to church, she no longer cooks or cleans much and only occasionally sews. She swings from bright, spinning cheer to black depression. But Dad adores her.

There is something animating her body, something that pulls us in, all of us. The sparking, sensuous current that runs between Mom and Dad must, I think, be at the center of what it means to be a wife.

Provo lies at the bottom of a bowl of hulking mountains. My childhood house sits at the foot of Y Mountain, painted with a white Y halfway to the summit. It's tradition—every year, students at BYU climb the mountain, armed with buckets for whitewashing the Y. Most are already winded when they get to our spot on the slope. You live here and mountains become backdrop, but every now and then you see them new again, unreasonably huge creatures ringing the valley. Growing up here, I heard them creak and shift at night. Belief in God comes easy with these omnipresent beings lurking over your shoulder. The mountains listen in on your secret thoughts, they judge your every move like the High Council, suited and tied and disapproving. Like them, the landscape talks in a man's voice, dry and stingy with greens, lawns a luxury, coaxed out of the soil only with constant drenchings. Our valley is unarguably male.

My family is a crowd. We are Dad and Mom, we are my sister Leda who is oldest, ten years ahead of me. Four brothers: Jonah, Luke, Jacob, Micah. I'm the youngest, and I am Amie. I will become Caitlin much later. We are loud, chaotic, Mormon.

Sunday mornings are cold cereal at the long wooden table, my brothers in a belching contest, faces sleep-creased, hair sticking up. Cold leaks in through our huge single-pane living room windows. I stand over the heat register, and hot air bellies up my nightgown, I put my hands lightly over the bulge.

Look, Leda. I'm pregnant, I say.

After breakfast my sister unrolls my pink sponge curlers, pulls a ringlet long, and together we watch it bounce into place. I put on my Sunday dress, hot pink taffeta trimmed with pink and white flowers. My sister's dress matches—hers short-skirted, mine long; she sewed them both. Mom emerges from her bedroom in a black slip over a bra over white garments, a halo of Chanel no. 5. She steps softly to the bathroom. Mom hasn't been to church in many weeks. She leans to wipe steam from the mirror, lips stretched over teeth while she mascaras her lashes. Sweat hurries down her face, licks her short hair into curls at her nape, and she blows out a gust of breath.

Time for my distemper shot, says Mom, laughing down at her mascara wand.

Distemper shot is what she calls hormone replacement. She had a hysterectomy shortly after I was born.

I'll remember you this way, Mom. One day when a hot flash rises through my body, eyeballs cooking in their sockets, I will see you again, leaning into your reflection, lace at the bottom of your black slip, bare feet on the bathroom floor. A drop of sweat runs down the side of your face and holds, shining, at the point of your chin.

Mom places her hands delicately on the bathroom counter as if to steady herself. She is balanced at a decision: church or no. She lifts her chin, turns her face to one side, flirting with her reflection. Church wins, today she will come with us.

As we load into the VW bus, Mom stops me with a hand on my shoulder. She licks her thumb and rubs my face clean.

Ew, Mom, I say. I hate the smell of her spit drying on my face.

You can't go to church looking like an urchin, she says.

At sacrament meeting we take up half a pew. Six kids makes us only a medium-size family in Provo. There are two twelve-child families in our neighborhood, and one with sixteen. One wife in each family, one woman constantly pregnant for over twenty years, pumping out child after child after child.

My hair gropes its way to Dad's suit and sticks to his sleeve, a blind, tentacled sea creature. He sweeps a hand down his arm to detach me, I make a whispering giggle and gather my hair behind, pin it against the back of the pew with my body. Micah draws mazes for me to solve; sacrament meeting is long and we are hungry and restless. I drag my pencil through my brother's maze while he draws another.

After church, the twelve-year-old deacons scramble outside to throw snowballs in the parking lot. A car pulls out of its parking space, crunching over snow, and my brother Luke crouches to grab the back bumper. The driver creeps down the road and Luke is pulled behind, slick Sunday shoes slide over icy streets, Luke in his dark suit and winter coat, tie flipping up and over his shoulder. A forbidden thrill, but irresistible to all the neighborhood boys. Dad doesn't notice.

I climb into the bus with the rest of the family, and Dad starts toward Cherry Lane.

Noooo, Dad! Micah and Jacob and Jonah and I all protest at once.

That's the old fogey way, says Jonah.

Stupid Sunday drivers, says Jacob.

What's wrong with old fogeys? I'm an old fogey, says Dad, waggling his eyebrows at us. But he's steering us in the other direction. We can see the slow march of cars going the old fogey way while we break free to the left, cheering. I am not convinced this route is faster, but my brothers have pronounced it so, and they know everything that I do not.

Oh Dad, says Leda. You're a young fogey.

They seem old to me, but Dad and Mom are still so young. Six kids and Dad isn't even forty yet.

At the mouth of Locust Lane, I see Luke ahead of us. He lets go of the bumper and slides on his shoes, wobbling, arms up. Dad is, as usual, oblivious; Mom has placed her fingertips over her closed eyes, crease growing between her brows.

Getting a headache? says Dad, soft now.

Mmmm, she says, mouth working like she's sucking on a candy.

Home is the smell of roast and church shoes kicked off savagely. Other families change out of their church clothes, but we eat in them and my brothers open their full mouths to show *see food*, then we do the dishes and roughhouse and spill gravy on our Sunday finery.

We rotate Sunday dinners between the six of us, one kid in charge of the whole shebang, roast and potatoes in the oven before church and dishes afterward. For a time, all six of us made Sunday dinner together and cleaned up together in a mad squirming knot in the kitchen. But we are too big, the kitchen too small, and Sunday dishes deteriorate into escalating, hostile games of Stop-touching-me/Not-touching-you as my brothers wrestle into the living room, booming the floor and shaking the house until Dad yells:

Simmer down!

And if it goes on, Dad boils down the hall, head gone deep red, jingling his belt buckle.

Blast!

Which is a terror-filled word from Dad, who does not swear. I don't know if he ever actually uses the belt or just threatens us with it. I will grow to think it would be a relief if he would use it, just get it over with.

Dinner is on the table, but church was too much. Mom has retreated to the dark of her bedroom where Dad brings her a plate. She turns over in bed toward him, devoting to Dad her last crumb of energy. The music is dead in her voice, it pulls low and slow from her center, each word a moan. Dad's answering tone is careful gentleness, the way you talk someone off a ledge.

This is normal. This is just how Mom is, on bad days. When she's in the bedroom with the door closed, you do not knock, you do not go in. She is like this for days or weeks or months, and then one day the door will open.

At night after a good day, Mom's laugh chimes, tumbles down the hall, Dad's answering laugh moving underneath.

Before school, Leda braids my hair. I fidget under her hands. Braiding takes hours, days, too long.

Play statue, says Leda.

I hold still, a statue.

Impossible, unbearable. I jiggle one knee. Both knees.

Come on. Statue, says Leda, pulling at a hank of hair.

I'm a statue picking flowers, I say. I swoop down to pick an imaginary flower, pulling my sister behind me, her hands full of hair. A statue doing an arabesque, I say. I am hilarious, I am genius, I am the most annoying of children.

Straight statue, says Leda, her patience wearing down. Be a statue of a soldier.

Straight statue, straight statue, straight and narrow is the path that leads to heaven.

There are days when Mom braids my hair. Mom sings to me:

Go to sleep my baby
Close your little eyes
The lady moon is watching
From out the dark'ling skies

Mom gets fanciful with my hair. She winds it into Princess Leia buns over each ear, before Princess Leia exists. When the movie comes out, Milo Moody at school will accuse me of being a copycat. Braids in double loops like a Swiss milkmaid. French braids and complicated braids of Mom's own invention crisscrossing and circling my head.

But most of the time, it's Leda. Leda teaches me camp songs, Leda pretends to pop one eyeball out of its socket, rolls it around in her mouth, pops it back in place, blinking open her eyes like she can see so much better now that her eyeball is clean. Leda is sixteen, old enough to date, and her boyfriends haunt the house and take her away from me, leave me alone with the brothers. I turn cartwheels for the boyfriend as he waits, I pirouette, tell silly stories, anything to hold his attention. Mom too. Mom charms Leda's boyfriends from bed, propped up on pillows. The boyfriend sits on the edge of the bed, laughing.

The phone rings. *Hello, Is Sister Myer there?*

Just a minute, I say. I hold the phone against my chest. Leda? I say. It's for Mom.

I'm so sorry, says Leda into the phone. Sister Myer is not available. May I take a message?

She hangs up the phone and bends down to face me. Okay, now you say it. *Sister Myer isn't available just now. May I take a message?*

Good. That way, says Leda, it's not a lie. You can't say she's not here. You say *unavailable*.

We are palace guards, keeping Mom safe inside the house inside her bedroom inside inside.

After school, Chrissie and I swing beside each other. Asphalt blurs beneath our feet. We pump our legs to get in sync.

Married! we say.

I try to keep us synced up but I wobble. I fall back as she shoots ahead.

Divorced, I say.

Nobody in our neighborhood is divorced. I have one aunt who is. And then my uncle, Mom's black-sheep brother. Before he dies, he will have been divorced seven times.

Chrissie was my very first friend in Provo. I was three when we moved here, and the day after our move, I climbed on the couch to look out the window at two girls walking up the hill hand in hand, one my age, one my sister's. I bounced in place until they rang the doorbell and that was it—at that age, proximity is all that's needed for a headfirst, all-consuming friendship, as intense as infatuation will be one day.

I laze in the swing and watch our toes make tracks in the frost on the black-top. Then Chrissie is up and running. I follow, a step behind, a beat slower than her. We live on the ragged edge of Provo, where a few scattered houses crawl up the toe of the mountain, scrub oak and sun-white rock. We are running up the steep of Apple Avenue when I slip and go down. Gravel-dirty snow reddens my hands, rocks studded into my knee. I open my mouth and cry, sitting on my bottom while melting snow wets my pants. Chrissie helps me up and I limp dramatically the rest of the way home. Chrissie is off to her house and me into mine, tears drying on my cheeks. Mom's bedroom door is closed. I touch it and know Mom is breathing on the other side. She is there in bed, Dad's big orange abstract-expressionist angel painting on the wall above. The angel flies headfirst, one hand raised in blessing, eyes lowered to Mom's dumb, dulled body. The angel's hand is blessing her. The hand is holding her down.

I want to knock but know I shouldn't. I lean my head against the door, listening through the wood for movement, voice, a Mom-shaped displacement of air. I've skinned my knee. I want Mom to kiss it better. That's what moms do, they kiss skinned knees better. And I have a memory or maybe it was a dream of Mom gathering me in her arms and saying, Oh poor baby. No, I do remember it. I remember my head between her breasts and her kiss on the part in my hair and all the soft mom of her holding me while I cry. But I can't remember when. I can't place it in time, or with a particular event. This is what is in my head, outside her bedroom door with the brown wood and gold-tone doorknob, and I know how to use a bobby pin to pick the lock, but that would be the exact wrong thing to do. If I wake her up, she won't be the mom who tucks her nose between my neck and shoulder to breathe me in. Her face will be pained, a line zipped between her eyebrows, and she will look at me with dull absence. I slide down the wall to sit and watch the blood bubble up on my knee.

Leda finds me at the end of the hall, my back against the linen closet. She helps me up, a finger held to her lips to shush me. In the bathroom she sets me on the counter, rubs at the knee with a rough washcloth. I try to cry quietly, Mom is just on the other side of the wall, but I'm not so good at that.

My brothers say I sound like a car shifting gears: WAAAAAH-haaaa-haaaa. Leda sweeps her dark hair over one shoulder and looks at me with an exaggerated pout, then wipes her hand upward over her face, revealing a bright smile underneath. Wipe down: pout. Wipe up: smile. I panic, fighting my breath, then pull on a smile to match hers, chest hiccuping with leftover sobs.

We're too much for Mom most days. My brothers, but especially my sister and me. If it wasn't for us, maybe she'd be well. I am sucking away my mother's life force simply by existing. All I have to offer is cheerfulness. The whole family needs it, Mom most of all. She bears the entire volume of our misery; the home cannot hold more. I am the youngest, I am sunny, it is my gift to jolly us all back to level, like my sister wiping her face into a smile.

Monday night is Family Home Evening. The church provides a lesson manual but ours goes largely unused.

Hey kids! yells my brother from the kitchen. Time for Family Home Draaag.

Most weeks it's a wrangle over division of housework, dinner, dishes. Someone will stomp off to their room in tears, yelling, You *Guys*!

Tonight is home movies. Mom appears from the hallway in her purple Peter Max caftan, blinking her black eyes back to life. We did okay today, we kept her safe and now she's up. We sit on the living room floor and Dad pulls the white blinds over our giant windows. My brother shuts off the light. Projector click-click-clicks and there's Mom on their honeymoon. They were fireguards, camping in the desert, the Shivwits Plateau. Dad had jury-rigged a washing machine that Mom worked with a treadle like a miniature seesaw. Onscreen she is all beauty queen bravado, red lipstick, cat-eye glasses, rolled jeans and knotted white shirt. Her feet in ballet flats rock the treadle.

If I were well, says Mom from the couch, You'd all be spoiled rotten.

Her voice loves these words, draws them out, *spoooiled rrrotten*. She would cook and clean and sew ruffles on my skirts, meet my father after work with a glass of lemonade (no cocktails for Mormons).

I'm leaning against my sister's legs, I feel her shift. A small, annoyed exhalation.

Mom as Donna Reed, Leda will say when we are grown, Not a chance.

Leda knew Mom in her more functional days, before her long slide into bed, before she got unsure at her edges, and even then she wasn't terribly interested in the domestic arts. Mom's black depression an excuse, then; or maybe her wish for a larger world was inverted, turned to despair. Punishment for wanting what wasn't meant to be hers. All of us, all the siblings, will suspect in our private moments that she malingers. That she has brought this on herself. Mom's illness has broken the celestial balance between husband and wife, her identity broken off from Dad's, taking monstrous shape behind her closed door. She is broken, and so Dad and the rest of us must pick up the slack.

Your wives will be so lucky, says Mom to the boys.

Other boys don't know how to cook or clean. When my brothers go on their missions at nineteen, they will be able to cook for themselves, not floundering and reduced to popcorn and canned soup like most young missionaries.

My sister and I are only doing what is expected, training for our wifely vocation. Of necessity we have skipped lessons, and so our home is lumpy and unfinished. We do not slice our sandwiches diagonally or sweep cobwebs from the ceiling. We do not wash our hands before dinner. There are things we don't know about homemaking that I won't even hear of until I'm grown. This harasses my sister who would have a clockwork home if she could, who will when she is married, blue-carpeted and squeaking with Ajax.

In the home movie, Dad shows how they measure rainfall, lifting the dipstick and grinning. He is already balding but handsome in his van Dyke beard.

Then the camera back in Dad's hands, and Mom laughs from behind her *Mad* magazine, waves her hand dismissively. *Oh stop*, she mouths.

Back then, possibilities spooled out in front of her, a thousand potential lives.

I've imagined a different life for Mom. One where she was free. No husband, no children. I try to imagine a world where I would never exist. She would have found power in her writing, I'm sure of it. Her poetry on shelves in libraries. This fantasy is so vivid I can see her striding a Paris street in flowing trousers, free and gloriously eccentric.

But that life was never available to her, not really. The story lived inside her as much as it lives in the world around us. She couldn't step outside the story, and though I've tried it's like jumping out of your own skin.

Mom the formidable poetess would have been seen as a monster. More, she would have seen herself as monstrous. And when her brain kicked off a bipolar storm—as it would, in no life could she escape the shocks that made her vulnerable, no scenario where her chemical makeup wouldn't be jostled to break—it would have been seen as evidence of her monstrosity.

She is crazy, people would think, she would think, because she thought she could make up a new story.

Mom comes home with a stylish scarf around her neck, lipstick, perfume. She's been at the bank. She stands in the entryway, red front door behind her, lights overhead like she's onstage. She tosses her hair back.

I have credit now, she says. Credit in my own name.

Until now it wasn't possible, a woman couldn't have credit without a husband or father's signature.

My brothers tell me a riddle: Okay, a boy and his father are in a car accident. The father dies instantly. The kid is put in an ambulance and taken to the hospital. The surgeon takes one look at the kid and says,

I can't operate on this boy! He's my son!

Who's the surgeon? my brothers ask.

This stumps me.

There is one grand evergreen in Kiwanis Park at the bottom of Apple Avenue, next to Wasatch Elementary School. With the first breath of spring, snow melted, Chrissie leads me up the branches where they are bare, close to the trunk, needles shielding us from the world outside. My legs are shaking, the ground far enough to squish me if I fall, but Chrissie is fearless. We perch inside the dark of the tree and Chrissie tries to teach me how to whistle through my cupped hands. I fail, and fail again, fail again.

~

Mom says she knew I was a dancer when I was six months old.

I was listening to a Herb Alpert album, she says, the one with the whipped cream on the cover? And you were in your Johnny Jump-Up, and I looked, and there you were, bouncing to the music! Just a coincidence, I said. But the record stopped and you stopped. And when I put on another record, you started up again, keeping perfect time.

Your first full sentence, she says, was, *I want to dance.*

I am going to be a prima ballerina, I am sure of this. Mom has already created my legend, my origin story, though I will eventually doubt that bit about my first sentence. I'm all in now. I have a pink picture book, *A Very Young Dancer*, perfect girl in perfectly done hair and leotard and tights. She is a fairy princess in the recital, and that will be me. I climb up the carpeted stairs to ballet class, a red star painted on the wall, red arrow pointing upward to stardom. The classroom ceiling leaks, and on rainy days the particleboard floor warps. The piano has dead keys, and I know by heart the pianist's favorite pieces when she hits the A above middle C with a click-thunk.

When I'm grown I'll learn that Dad paid for my lessons with artwork. No money for ballet, but the ballet mistress has a gallery of Dad's work, her walls crowded with figure studies.

After class I take my hair out of its ballet bun, it stands up and back from my face in wide waves. I step from the bathroom down the hall to Mom's room. She is sitting up in bed and I bring her my day, the world outside her bed, the people I've met, characters at school, at ballet class. I dance the choreography we learned today: pas de chat, pas de chat, pas de bourrée.

Come here, Ultra Violet, she says. Let me see your wild hair.

Ultra Violet. I know who she is, I know she is part of Andy Warhol's Factory. Nobody else in Provo knows who Ultra Violet is, or even Andy Warhol.

I already know that I don't fit in at school. Chrissie is my shield, my bodyguard, my proof of legitimacy. By myself I'm all wrong. I wear the peach pantsuit Leda made with grass embroidered on the hem of the pants and a flower growing from the jacket pocket. Too colorful for Happy Valley, too modern, too experimental. Not quiet like the neighbors' handmade clothes, plain blouses, simple skirts. Not fresh-from-the-store like the rich kids further up the mountainside, their Peter Pan collars and crisp jeans.

(Maybe Mom made the pantsuit. She is good with a sewing machine and more eccentric than Leda, but her projects taper off as her sickness grows.)

We can't afford new clothes; it's hand-me-downs or my sister's creations done up on the sewing machine.

The brothers are tall in the kitchen, their legs a forest of blue jeans. I've gotten out of bed in my white nightgown, the waves of laughter and music from the stereo finally unbearable. I'm missing out on all the fun. I've been carried here on their voices and I'm in love with all of them, warmed in kitchen light, dark night massed outside our living room windows.

You're supposed to be in bed, says Jonah.

Please, I say. I grab his hands and put my feet on his.

Okay, okay, he says.

We dance, my feet on his, and I'm bursting open with happiness.

We live in Utah Valley but my brothers sarcastically call it Happy Valley. The church enjoins us to be in but not of the world; we are *in* but not *of* Utah. We make a distinction between Mormon and Utah Mormon. You can be Mormon and be an artist like Dad, you can be Mormon and a poet like Mom, but these collisions are suspect in Happy Valley. Even more suspect is Mom sealed up in her bedroom, rarely attending church.

I wish I could go to sacrament meeting, she will say. Already I hate the martyred face she makes, held stiff as if too much movement will crack it.

But she wants to be well, or she wants to want to be well. She wants to eat the Wonder Bread embodiment of Christ, drink the water in little paper cups standing in for His blood. She wants us to know it's not her fault. She feels left out of church the way I feel left out after my bedtime while the brothers stay up late.

The brothers give me a glass of water, push me back toward bed. Like Mom I'm trapped here in my room, floating in lonely dark.

I'm home from school with a stomachache, propped up in bed with a book open on my knees but I can't read. I close my eyes and hear the mountains behind our house whisper, one to the other. Mom calls me from the doorway and I drag myself out of bed, book falling to the floor. She ushers me into her bathroom to give me an enema. She is forceful and efficient with the tube. She is intimate with violent cures; we're going through this ordeal together on the bathmat. I sit on the toilet, naked from the waist down, my feet dangling above the floor. I'm folded over my stomach and crying. Shit explodes out of me like a confetti cannon on the fourth of July. I don't yet know the word *shit*, and we don't use the word *poop*. I can't remember what word my family uses for the substance jackhammering the toilet water. I cry louder, mouth open. I want her to know how miserable this is.

She knows. She administers enemas to herself, too. Before her death, her body will have been sliced open several times. Already her uterus is gone. Years from now her gall bladder will follow and her stomach will be sewed down to the size of a coin purse. She will have screws installed in her ankles. Electrodes fastened to her head and current shocked through her limbs. She will go on juice fasts and diet shakes and stuff herself with herbal potions. She will get Heavy, then Skinny, then Heavy, and Skinny again. She will turn herself in front of a bank of full-spectrum lights like a chicken on a rotisserie. And she will take drugs to even out her moods, drugs to lift her depression, drugs to focus her attention, wake her up, put her to sleep, to offset the side effects of the other drugs, drugs to prevent seizures and aphasic episodes or maybe the drugs will cause aphasia or seizures. She will shake when a dose is late, or she will be unable to assemble a coherent sentence. She will panic if Dad is unable to refill a prescription, eyes gone opaque, black with fear.

But that's later. For now her pharmacopeia is manageable.

Mom has allowed me the rare privilege of climbing into her bed while Dad gets the consecrated oil from the fridge. It's olive oil. Nobody in Utah cooks with olive oil, not in 1974. Like everyone else in town, our only bottle has been blessed and waits congealed in the fridge for occasions like today. Mom stands by while Dad warms the bottle in his hands, tips a few drops onto the part in my hair. He puts his hands heavy on my head and prays, blesses me to be well.

He is halfway through the *Amen* when I make a dash for the bathroom to throw up in the toilet.

I stand on shaking legs in the doorway of the bathroom and Mom claps her hands, laughing.

That was a quick answer! I bet you feel a lot better now.

I nod, wobbling down the hall to my room. Mom poaches eggs in milk for me, milk soaking into a thick slice of homemade wheat bread and drizzled with honey, my favorite sick-day food.

Was it Mom? Or had I already learned how to poach the eggs myself? I can't be sure.

By bedtime I'm violently sick, vomiting into our big stew pot next to the bed. I throw up until there's nothing left, fall asleep with my head hanging off the edge of the bed over the pot. I wake in the middle of the night to a hallucination, my hands huge as oven mitts. I crawl out of bed, skirt the pot full of vomit on the floor.

Mom and Dad's room is at the end of the hall. I spirit the door open as silently as I can.

They sleep spooned at the far edge, next to the window. In front of Mom is an expanse of king-size bed. The room stretches impossibly wide, bed receding in space, it will take me hours to cross the carpet. I want to burrow into bed with them, feel Mom curl around me, warm and safe, the smallest spoon.

Mom? I say.

Mom turns over to face Dad, murmurs his name. Dad sits up.

Your mother needs her sleep, he says.

I'm hallucinating, I say.

She'll have to get out of bed now, I think. This is serious. She'll have to put her cool hand on my forehead, she'll have to make it better.

Go back to bed, he says. I'll be there in a minute.

I close the door behind me, toes clutching carpet, the hallway lengthening away from me. I put a hand to the wall to guide me back to my room, crawl into bed, an island in the middle of the warping house.

The hall light flips on. My sister appears, an animated stick figure in the light from the doorway.

Leda puts me in the bath to get my fever down. Bright bathroom light bounces hard and loud off porcelain. She wraps me up in a towel and gets Dad to carry me back to bed. I hug myself with my arms, shrink into a ball under the covers.

Behind our house, to the east, is the Wasatch Range. At the west end of the city, on the far side of Utah Lake, the Oquirrh Mountains. They look blue from our living room windows: three windows facing south, three open to the west, Provo spilling down the slope below us. We sit down to dinner as sun slips behind the Oquirrhs, and we applaud the colors painted across the sky.

We have no lawn. We have boulders. We have a slim tree we plant in a bed of rocks, and my sister tells me it will one day be as tall as the house. This does me no good. Except that evergreen at the park, there are no climbable trees nearby, and it will take twenty-five years for the new tree to grow that big. I try to imagine living that long, to the terrible old age of thirty. I'll surely be dead by then, or married, which to a kid looks like an ending. I'm anticipating marriage, but happily ever after in fairy tales is the end of the story.

Did you wash your hands? says Chrissie.

I'm stepping out of the bathroom, toilet flushing behind me. I hold up my hands for us both to see.

They're pretty clean, I say.

You're supposed to wash your hands after, she says. She looks ceilingward as if to ask Heavenly Father how I got so stupid.

At Chrissie's house, we eat salted apples her mother has sliced, neat little wedges where the core was. Chrissie's mom has dusky circles under her eyes; she's given birth to six daughters. She looks tired but makes the house so orderly I don't know where to put my hands. Blue carpet and blue-edged china and a picture of blue-eyed Jesus in prayer. There are baby circles under Chrissie's eyes to match her mom's, arterial blue.

Her little sister Betsy wants to play with us but Chrissie shuts it down.

We don't play with babies, she says.

Betsy's arms are straight by her sides and she stands there openfaced and starts to cry.

Kindergarten baby / growing in the gravy, we sing, as snot and tears run down Betsy's face. We're out of the house before she can stick herself to us. Chrissie winds up and is running full-speed by the time I'm at the front step. We go headlong into the field, weeds slapping at us. She stumbles but will not allow herself to fall, I know she won't stop until my breath is shrieking out of me, until I fall down and yell after her.

We stay out until Chrissie's mom calls from the doorway, dinnertime. It's getting dark when I slam into the house, our red door shuddering behind me. Dinner is a favorite: frazoline, elbow macaroni and hamburger and cheese and whatever else is leftover thrown into a pot. I lean over my food and a bright drop of blood splashes the white plate.

Gross! says a brother.

I bring my hand quick to my nose; it's sprung a gusher of blood. During World War II, Mom got nosebleeds. Eleven years old and her nose gushed, the front of her blouse soaked red in seconds. Her doctor prescribed Jell-O water, and Mom got first crack at the town's entire ration of Jell-O whenever it came in.

I run to the bathroom, twist a plug of toilet paper and stuff it into my nostril. It soaks through, wet bloodclump, and I switch it out, again and again. I will become used to this gesture—nosebleeds will follow me into high school, and I will have a standing excuse to leave class when blood tracks down my lip.

Mom? I'm standing in the doorway of the bedroom. My nose won't stop bleeding, I say.

Make some Jell-O water. Her voice comes out of the dark.

How?

Just like you're making regular Jell-O, but don't put it in the fridge. You have to drink it down warm before it sets up. Pick any flavor you want, Sweetie. Her voice grows weight. I hear her body shift, she is already sliding back into sleep.

There's only red in the cupboard. It feels like cherry-flavored blood going down my throat.

Saturday morning, the bedroom door is open, sunlight shines into the hallway from the window. We all pile into bed with Mom and Dad, and she says, This is why we wanted a king-size bed, so we could all fit. Her eyes are shining crescents. All six of us kids have the same eyes, almost disappearing when we smile. She buries her nose into Micah's blond hair, her youngest son and everyone's favorite, and he laughs and squirms.

She pulls Jacob close on her other side. Sponge babies, she says, are always the sweetest.

She is talking about the birth control she was using when Jacob was conceived, when I was conceived. He and I were sweet babies, and we are sweet children. Jacob of all the brothers is nicest to me, though Micah and I are closest.

Although I can't articulate it, I know already that sweetness is more important in a girl than in a boy; it's what I have going for me.

I am sweet and I am cheerful and I stay where I am, but I want to crawl over my brothers' bodies, squeeze in beside Mom. I want to burrow my head into her guts. I want to pry open her lips, stuff my hands in her mouth, I want to print her smiling face on my insides, place her in me like a moon, smiling and smiling until I'm stuffed overfull with her. I want to own her. I want to obliterate her.

After Dad's pancakes, it's Bugs Bunny and Roadrunner on TV, and after *Land of the Lost*, it's time for me to make bread.

I scoop wheat to feed the electric wheat grinder on the countertop. The grinder is mine. I was in a commercial for Magic Mill wheat grinders at six years old, and they paid me with my very own electric wheat grinder. It roars like a motorcycle engine and wheat clangs and rattles down its throat. It jumps and jitters across the counter and unplugs itself in excitement. The motor winds down, dies. I plug it back in and try to hold on while it revs up, but I'm stumbling along the counter to keep up. Finally I let go and watch it jank around.

Bread making takes hours. I love the feeling of a dough in my hands, like the firm bottom of a fat baby. I love to punch down the sponge in the bowl after the first rising, feel it sigh and collapse around my hand.

We have enormous red-topped canisters of whole wheat around the house that we use as end tables. Mormons are commanded to keep a two-year supply of food, stocked up against the Last Days. We have jars of preserves on big wooden shelves downstairs, water in mason jars, and wheat.

My swarm of brothers elbow each other to get the first hot slice as it comes out of the oven. The smell blooms from the kitchen to fill the house. Butter and honey shine, melted into my own thick slice.

Look, says Chrissie.

She's levered a rock out of the dirt. Underneath an oasis of darker earth, alive with glossy black creatures.

Potato bugs, she says.

She takes my hand and drops one into my palm. It curls into a shining ball. She rubs her nose, leaves a loamy black smudge between nostril and lip.

Chrissie lifts another rock with a stick and something moves out of the dark, sends an electric shock up the middle of my spine before my brain can even name the creature. Tarantula.

My fear of spiders is utter, tangled with awe. I can't even scream. I'm standing without knowing how I got to my feet.

The spider is on its toes, swaying. Chrissie leans forward from the waist, stick in hand, brushes the dirt just in front of it. It steps sideways, foot foot foot foot.

A vicious tremor travels down my body. I'm behind her now, my hands on the wings of her shoulder blades. Chrissie holds her arm out and back to protect me. She keeps her body between me and the spider.

My siblings and I keep the house from descending entirely into filth, if only barely, only by our fingernails. Other families say *chores*, but we say *jobs*. It's *restriction*, not *grounding*. Dad exhausts himself trying to marshal us to our jobs, now stalking the house for Saturday inspection. He is head of the family like Christ is head of the church; today he is a stand-in for Jesus, making sure my room is Saturday Clean. There's a primary song:

Saturday is a special day.
It's the day we get ready for SUN-day!
We clean the house and we wash our clothes.
That's how we get ready for SUN-day!

My brothers prance up and down the hall singing in falsetto while Dad examines my bedroom. He runs a finger along the top of my bedroom door, his half-tongue-in-cheek, white-glove check. If I fail inspection today, I'm on restriction for the week. Dad lowers his voice in a faux-disciplinarian timbre.

Well, it'll have to do, he says, mock-glowering at me.

Then he sees the pile of dress-ups in the corner. Blood washes up into his scalp. He gets quiet, a shift from hilarious to terrifying in three one-thousandths of a second. I'm in trouble and he doesn't have to say a word.

Saturday night Leda rolls my hair into pink sponge curlers before bed. I sleep all night on a nest of plastic curlers for Sunday morning ringlets.

I walk to Chrissie's house for our race down Apple Avenue to school. I ring the bell and her mother answers the door. She is tall, broad-shouldered, with the body of an aging athlete, hot-rollered Mom hair. She does not smile.

Chrissie's sick, she says. She can't come to school.

This has never happened before. Chrissie doesn't get sick. I do. I get every flu, I get high fevers and hallucinations, I throw up and have daylong stomachaches. Chrissie isn't sick like that. This isn't sick like Mom, where she's sick and then fine and then sick and then fine. This is sick as plot point. The kind of sick where the heroine has a cough in the first act. As everyone knows, in plays and stories, a cough is never just a cough.

Very quickly, Chrissie is in the hospital, and I'm carrying a grubby construction paper card from Mrs. Steed's class to Chrissie's house. We all drew hearts and wrote *Get Well!!* in crayon.

Her family gets to see her in the hospital, even her little sister Betsy who tells me how Chrissie's hair was all tangled from being in bed so long. I ask Leda if I can go too, but she shakes her head at me, her face grave.

You're too young, she says.

But Betsy gets to go, I say.

Betsy's family, says Leda. Hospital rules. Sorry, Squeaky.

I am Squeaky because I squeak when I laugh, but now I shrug at Leda, trying not to cry. It isn't fair, I say.

At family prayer we kneel around the bed, leaning on our elbows. I close my eyes hard and Dad's deep voice makes colors on my brainscreen, dark purple and maroon to match his dark voice in the black of family prayer.

If it be Thy will, prays Dad, please bring healing to Chrissie.

Make her better, I pray in my head. I send the words up into the black, riding under Dad's, pale scratches. Make her better. Make her better.

Does Heavenly Father answer our prayers? I ask Mom.

Always, she says. She opens her mouth and pauses, looks at me.

Just, sometimes, she says, the answer is No.

After a few weeks we stop asking for Chrissie to get better at family prayer. The prayer becomes:

Father, please be with Chrissie and her family through this difficult time.

~

Chrissie has acute leukemia, and nobody tells me there is no getting better. I hear it as *cute* leukemia, which of course makes sense (Chrissie's cuteness her undoing).

It's Saturday, and I'm sleeping in. I wake up and my father is sitting on my bed. His face is a hard slap. I'm sure I've done something terribly wrong, I'm in bad trouble.

Chrissie died, he says.

I shake my head at him.

I react almost too fast, panicked, sudden howl, face open, hands open and grabbing at the air like an infant.

Later that day, it falls out of my head. I am playing jump rope, practicing the crossed arms and double jump, Chrissie and I are champion jump-ropers. Playing and laughing, and then I look up and my brother Jacob is looking at me, grim. It is a violence, that face, and I remember. This time I have done something very bad, maybe unforgivable. Laughing on the day she died. It wasn't just a light laugh, either. It was one of those hilarious, all-consuming, out-of-control kid laughs.

I bend over, holding my stomach. Chrissie is dead and I am grotesque.

The Aughts

FUNERAL RITES BELONG TO WOMEN in Mormonism. In the old days women washed and dressed the body. Morticians do that now, but women take care of the rest. I don't remember anything after the funeral, after leaning into Chrissie's coffin to see her one last time, but the Relief Society ladies must have made ham and funeral potatoes. We must have gathered in the church cultural hall, paper plates loaded down, little kids in our Sunday shoes clicking on varnished floor.

Leda and I do our part for Mom's arrangements, meet with the mortician to work out the details. The gravesite must be lined with concrete, then steel. This is state law, we are told. Because of the embalming chemicals.

We are going over these details, measuring the budget, and Leda sucks in a breath.

I just remembered, when I was a teenager, she says. Mom told me something she wanted for her funeral.

It was a Fourth of July parade. They were watching the parade when a horse-drawn hearse clopped by, the back filled with red, white, and blue flowers. Mom saw it and said:

That's what I want for my funeral. A Black Mariah.

Is that even possible, says Leda now.

The mortician looks like a mortician from Central Casting. Pale and pudgy, bad tan suit. But he laughs with us when we laugh. He looks cheerful and interested at the thought of a Black Mariah.

Let me make some calls, he says.

We sit with him while he calls around, finds a funeral home with a Black Mariah they're willing to rent out, horses included. The Black Mariah was built for older caskets. It won't fit a modern metal casket. But we've already chosen a simple poplar box, narrow enough for the carriage. We remembered poplars grew at the ranch. The newer, deluxe caskets are in terrible taste. Brushed steel, pink-washed, or blue-washed casket. I don't know what it's supposed to resemble, what model of luxury this is meant to emulate.

Poplar looks good to both of us, and has the virtue of being cheaper. It is terribly expensive to bury a corpse, and Mormons don't believe in cremation. Our actual bodies will be resurrected and perfected in the Last Days, they say. Of course Heavenly Father is capable of restoring a body that was burned to cinders, but the implication is that it would be impolite to make Him go to the extra work if it isn't necessary.

Two of the brothers stop by on their morning run. Here we are in the mortuary, my brothers in shorts and running shoes, sweating, making rank puns about burying the hatchet and making no bones about it. It's us, the volume turned up, up close and big as life. We want an Addams Family–style Fourth of July parade for Mom—we'll dress Dad up in a coachman's hat and tails, with the whole procession of cars hung up behind a horse-drawn carriage down the mountain and through the middle of Provo. Everyone else can go around us, this is our moment.

1975

RUNNERS PAUSE AT THE CORNER of our hill. It's already a steep hike to our house. But the road leading past the house and to the trail up the mountain is a grade in its own class. The runners pause, hands on hips. They breathe hard and look at the trail, pace, work themselves up.

I want to stay a minute in that evergreen tree in the park with Chrissie. Rub my hands together and shape them into a hollow. She shows me how to leave a vent at the bottom, how to flutter the tone by lifting a finger, two fingers, all four fingers. Spit runs down my palms and nothing. She tries a new tack, then—a basic whistle, lips pursed. Her whistle trills and swoops. Her thin hair sticks to a branch, I can see the shape of her skull underneath. I purse my lips and it's nothing but spit-wet air.

Childhood is the kingdom where nobody dies / Nobody that matters, that is, writes Edna St. Vincent Millay.

You'll see her again, says Leda, brushing my hair. She's waiting for you in the Celestial Kingdom.

Chrissie was so righteous she didn't have to live long enough to be baptized. Instead she gets to skip directly to heaven, where she rolls endlessly on a vast lawn with my family's dead pets; my great-grandfather, his amputated leg regrown and mouth full of his own teeth; my great aunt, cured of cerebral palsy and free of her wheelchair. Chrissie is already out of my reach, already sitting in judgment over me, answering me with silence when I say her name, calling her over and over.

I have to stay here on earth, the kingdom of childhood already closing behind me. I have to grow up, I have to sin. I will have to know more of the world than I ever wanted, will be in the world and of the world, sin and corruption blossoming outward from my core.

Until.

First wiving.
    Wife: seven-year-old girl.
    Husband: teenage boy, a cousin.
    Year: 1975. The girl wears red-white-and-blue shorts.
    Place: her home, the basement family room. Sunlight shines in through a sliding glass door, stripes the yellow and orange shag carpet.
    Consummation: the boy is watching TV, invites the girl to sit on his lap. He takes her hand and places it first on his belly. They both watch the TV screen, they watch but don't see. He opens his shorts and moves her hand millimeter by millimeter, wraps her hand around his penis. Silky skin, hard and hot underneath, his hand on top of hers.
    Duration: a few seconds, thirty seconds, a minute, an hour.
    Their bodies fit, his chest against her back her bottom his hips their legs. A flood of love and shame. She knows she has done something wrong. Soon she will be eight years old. She will be baptized into the Church of Jesus Christ of Latter-day Saints, and will then be fully responsible for all of her actions. When she is baptized, she will be immersed in water and made clean of all her sins. She suspects this sin, however, might be etched too deep for water.

Not *her*. Me. I am the girl on my cousin's lap. Do not mistake.

~

A memory hangs in my head. I'm eight, I've been baptized. My cousin in boxer shorts on an unmade bed. Gap open at the crotch. This picture is unconnected, swinging loose. I don't know what comes before or after. All I know is a slippery feeling of habit.

In the bible, the story of Yael and Sisera is told twice. Sisera was commander of the Canaanite army. On losing the Battle of Mount Tabor, Sisera took shelter in Yael's tent, believing that she, like her husband Heber's tribe, was an ally.

> *Then Jael Heber's wife took a nail of the tent, and took an hammer in her hand, and went softly unto him, and smote the nail into his temples, and fastened it into the ground: for he was fast asleep and weary. So he died.*
>
> (JUDGES, CHAPTER 4:21, *HOLY BIBLE*)

In the next chapter, Yael becomes a song:

> *Blessed above women shall Jael the wife of Heber the Kenite be, blessed shall she be above women in the tent.*
>
> *He asked water, and she gave him milk; she brought forth butter in a lordly dish.*
>
> *She put her hand to the nail, and her right hand to the workmen's hammer; and with the hammer she smote Sisera, she smote off his head, when she had pierced and stricken through his temples.*
>
> *At her feet he bowed, he fell, he lay down: at her feet he bowed, he fell: where he bowed, there he fell down dead.*
>
> (JUDGES, CHAPTER 5: 24–27, *HOLY BIBLE*)

A story can be turned in your hand, seen from behind, above, below. It looks different whichever way you turn it.

Seven years old.

I wear my hair in two long braids.

My sister braids my hair, she pulls it tight when I fidget and whine.

I am seven and my arms and legs are tender as new grass.

I stuff bread crusts behind the piano.

I pick boogers from my nose, stick them to my bedroom wall.

I am perfect and horrible the way all seven year olds are perfectly horrible.

Every seven year old in all the history of the world is perfect as a bead of water held and trembling on the side of a cup.

I am seven and I climb into my cousin's lap.

I love him the way I love all the big boys, the almost-men who rumble through my house.

He takes my hand and sunlight rushes up and through my body.

My body flares and my spirit bows, at our feet it bows, it bows and falls at our feet.

I open my mouth and swallow this whole, my cousin and his hot skin, me and my hand and the singing thrill that moved through my body. It's nothing, it is not part of my story, I slip it into a pocket behind my ribs and go on with school and dance class and recital and booming racket of brothers and I will not notice that my story has fragmented, exploding outward into the sky above Happy Valley.

Other stories will be brighter in my memory. In the long closet at school, Lisa who is not exactly my friend and I pull down our pants, we show each other our parts, hairless and tucked away.

Another school friend lets me watch him pee, sparkling arc into a patch of scrub oak.

My shame sparks and then dulls as I get older. We were only curious kids, only doing what kids do.

The story with my cousin will be wrapped up and hidden. I will come to believe it's a perverse dream. It settles deeper than other stories, the way smoke blackens a lung.

This isn't an unusual story. This story is happening in a thousand thousand homes to young humans. It is nothing at all. It is what happens when sex is squeezed into a box and giftwrapped for people who don't know any different, who have been trained from birth to think it was always theirs. Once you believe some humans should by nature, through gender or skin or *difference*, occupy a lower, more limited place in the world, once you believe they owe you their love, their attention, their obeisance, it leaks into everything, and this has been the story since the first story was written.

In family lore, Mom's depression began postpartum, after my third brother Jacob was born. But it was seeded much earlier.

Mom's first child died in her womb at six months. She had to carry him to term. She had to give birth to a dead baby.

And then she went on to birth six more. This would unhinge anyone.

She was finished having kids after my last brother was born. Her body had given birth six times, more than enough.

And then I came along.

Maybe her illness was born earlier, grew from the blood-fertilized ground at Mountain Meadows, where early Mormons slaughtered a whole wagon train of settlers. Mountain Meadows, the land my great-grandfather bought after the massacre, the land beneath my grandfather's scrubby little ranch, tiptoed by scorpions between rows of squash. Mountain Meadows, where Mom grew up and baled hay beside her father, her world bounded by the red cliffs between St. George and Cedar City.

Or her sickness sprouted from above-ground nuclear tests upwind of their ranch. Mom and her family and all the town went outside to watch the cloud bloom out over the desert; white ash carried on the wind and dusted their shoulders as high school cheerleaders shook their pompoms for the USA.

And then the sheep died.

And then Mom's first baby died.

And then, and then.

I was wrong. My *Until* wasn't on my cousin's lap. Not there, not at the edge of Chrissie's casket. You have to go further back, throw a line to my mother's *Until*, before I was born. My *Until* prefigured in hers—she was a different woman, would have been a different mother before she gave birth again, again, again. Before the corpse of her first child floated in her womb.

Before she became a wife, when she was dating the young man who would become Dad, she spent a summer working in New York City. She and her friend, Skin, fresh to the big city from Utah.

We called her Skin because she was skinny, says Mom.

The nickname sounds clever and dashing to me.

They went to their first real New York party, the place packed with Julliard and Princeton grads.

In her journal, Mom wrote: *The refreshments were liquid, + plentiful. I nursed a glass of ginger ale all evening. The conversation was carried on several feet above my left eyebrow, but I was assured that it was both stimulating + witty.*

A young man tried his best to flirt with the Utah girls.

"Wouldn't you like me to seduce you?"

"No."

"Don't boys ask you questions like that back in Utah or Arizona or wherever you're from?"

"No."

"What is this place called you're from?"

Skin sat a little straighter, folded her hands demurely in her lap + began in a small voice: "I'm from a little town on the border of Utah & Arizona. It's called Short Creek."

"Isn't that the place where they practice . . ."

"Oh no, we don't just practice," Skin continued. "It is for real. That's why we're here, you see."

Lover boy: "What's why you're here?"

"Well, because we weren't just practicing, of course. You see, when Aunt Matilda (she's our Sister Wife) found out the law was coming, she coaxed dear Brother Amos Jessop (he's our husband) to let us leave. She wanted us to see how the world lives so we'd know."

"Go on, know what?"

"Like the Bible says, out in the world the men are all beasts, so we'd be glad to come back to dear Brother Amos Jessop, even if he is so old."

"Ummm," Lover Boy answered dully. "And how old is your husband?"

"Oh he's 78 years old, but he's not a leering prancing goat like the Bible says the men of the world are."

If Mom had held to her sharp-witted self, if she had dared to step outside her small Mormon universe, she might not have given birth seven times. She might not have married. And I would never have existed at all. My *Until*, then, only the moment of birth.

There is beauty all around
When there's love at home;
There is joy in ev'ry sound
When there's love at home.

I am cast in a short ballet, my costume a yellow dress, petticoated and swiss-dotted. Onstage I dance with my pretend father, mother, brother.

Making life a bliss complete
The hymn moves us across the floor—
When there's love at home.

At home, real home, I make fun of the impossibly perfect family, the drippy, sappy hymn, but my heart goes sick at the refrain, this mother who holds me close, releases me to run full-tilt where Father waits on one knee, arms out to either side to catch my brother and me. My real family does not even exist in the same universe as my stage family. I used to be part of a *we*, a Myer among Myers, my brothers loud and heedless as wild dogs, my sister too-perfect, but they were mine and I was theirs. Now I'm something else, an *I*, drifting from the family shore. Onstage I jump and spin in the air to land, sitting, on Father's arm. I'm not much of a ballerina yet but I give myself over to the dance, delirious fantasy, run and jump again and again, I could live in rehearsal, live on this lighted stage floating in the dark, looming curtains and ceiling as distant as the Celestial Kingdom.

Run and spin and jump and I overshoot, flip backward over Father's arm and land headfirst on the hollow stage floor. The boom fills the empty theater, repeats in my head. Boom and I wrench myself to standing. Boom the director asks if I'm okay. Boom I say okay, okay, let's go again. Arms and legs shaking, fantasy gone dumb, I set my face and run and spin and brake too soon, land on my feet before Father's waiting arm. I try over and over again, willing myself to trust the turn, trust the strong arm of the father. I miss as many times as I land right. In the performance I am sick with terror and leap anyway. I grab at his shoulder to steady myself, and he pulls to standing while I balance on his arm.

When I have to give back the yellow dress, I lock myself in my room and cry.

My brother is tickling me. I fold up, collapse onto the floor, and he's on top of me.

Stop. Stop! I say.

I'm laugh-crying.

STOP!

He doesn't stop. I'm laughing but tears run sideways into my ears, an angry laugh. Pure hot girl rage. I get his hand in my mouth and bite down. When he lets go, I make my nails into claws, rake at his face. I shout, joyfully monstrous.

He covers his face and jumps to his feet, a loud suck of breath.

We're both shocked to quiet. Only a few seconds. Then he turns deep red and roars:

You *bit* me!

I see disbelief in his face, panic. I see humiliation.

I didn't know I had that power.

The moment is unbearable for both of us, violates everything we think we know about the world. I'm sick with embarrassment, my loss of control.

I can never, never use this power again. My brothers boom the living room floor as they wrestle, they give me Indian burns and suspend me over the stairwell threatening to drop me, they pull my hair and hold me down for water torture, and if I cry they call me a wuss. But my violence is too serious.

They don't mean what they do.

I do.

My rage has to be reserved for real danger. Kidnapper-with-a-knife danger. I don't know yet that the border is porous and shifting. I can't know I'll mistake threat for misunderstanding, for love, for anything else.

They're only boys, they can't help themselves.

My mother's long fingernail is in my ear. My head is in her lap, and she is dragging a perfectly manicured nail through the paths and folds of my ear. My eyes are closed, body blissed.

All clean, says Mom.

Don't stop, I say, not moving my head.

There's nothing left to clean. Perfect, pink, little shell-like ears, she says.

Please, I say.

She indulges me. All the wax gone, nail scrapes bare skin, my hands tight between my knees, she digs in deep. It hurts but I don't want her to stop. I picture the red trail she leaves. She leans down and whispers:

You came out of my womb flirting with the doctor who delivered you.

It's a half-joke. Delivered gently, but her voice is thick.

I sit up and the air feels colder for the warmth I've left. I don't know how old I am. Has she always said this, or does she smell my corruption, do I stink of my cousin's skin?

Mom says: Your first time on an airplane, I gave all you kids Dramamine to put you to sleep, but instead you and Micah were wired, running up and down the aisles. I found you, she says, sitting on a man's lap, flirting like crazy.

I remember this. I remember the fat white man and I remember lying about my age, holding up three fingers although I was only two. My back fit against his belly, his lap warm. My character formed at birth, already evident in toddlerhood. Mom sees right into my perverted little heart.

But what does a two-year-old know about flirting? Maybe I was only fearless. I believed I could be friendly to anyone. And then and also: I am wrong and I am a flirt. Derrick Wolf raised his hand at school to complain that I touched him. The boys my age are repulsed by me and my cooties, but I like boys, and maybe I shouldn't, not so much.

I am supposed to grow up to be a wife. I am supposed to attract a righteous man. I am built for, meant for wiving. I will be to my husband as the church is to Jesus. I am meant to please him.

But I am already wrecked.

Flirting is shameful except when it isn't. When Mom flirts it isn't serious, she's just playing at it with my sister's boyfriends, they fall in love with her like everyone else but harmlessly—she's a mom and a wife and so above the mess of my need.

Her earnest flirtation is saved for Dad. She goes to bed early and Dad says: Don't start without me.

He raises his eyebrows at her, cartoonishly suggestive.

Mmm, better hurry then, says Mom, swinging her hips as she goes.

On another day, Mom is up, her liveliest self. Jacob is fresh from the shower and she chases him, threatening to snatch the towel from around his waist. They circle the stairwell madly, laughing and shouting, Mom gains on him, fingers reaching, and the towel slips from his hips, hangs swinging from her hand.

Jacob pounds down the stairs to his room in a flash, yelling, Moooooom! The rest of us freeze in place. She wasn't meant to actually win. Mom's cheeks go pink, a laugh burbles up from her belly, bounces high off the ceiling.

Can I sleep over at Jennifer's house? I ask.

Ask your mother, says Dad.

I step apologetically into the bedroom.

You have your father wrapped around your little finger, says Mom. You're his princess, he'd do anything for you.

She says to ask you, I say to Dad.

We'll see, he says.

Next time I'll tell him she said yes.

You're his little princess, says Mom. I feel her bitterness, but can't name it.

Once upon a time, Eve was created to fill a man's need. She sprang from his rib but wasn't free, she was hooked to him, defined by him, her daughters' destiny written at the beginning of the world. The woman's reason for being centers on the man. She is his companion, his caretaker; above all she offers him safety between her legs.

This is the story behind and under every story we know. There are other founding myths but they all mean the same, that the woman exists for the use of the man.

It's also an aspirational story, one I'm being raised to love. The woman awakened—to herself, to the world—by a kiss. A woman gains status, substance when she becomes a wife. We are all part of the story, men and women, all held inside its borders.

Q: What does it look like, outside the story?

A: Loneliness.

1976

THE SUMMER OF MY EIGHTH birthday, I am in the far back of the VW Bus, cozy in blankets and pillows on top of suitcases. Leda rides shotgun, Dad drives, brothers on the bench seats in the middle. A road trip to Dad's parents' farm in Pennsylvania. Mom is at home—she's ghostwriting a book, but she likely spends most days sealed up in her room, sunk into the depths of her bed. That isn't fair. She will finish the book, *Own Your Own Body*.

When I'm grown I'll laugh, hearing the *fuck you* of that title for the first time. Mom's body forever slipping free of her hands like a live fish, she tried to pummel it into submission, but your body is yourself and the submission was hers.

But now she has stayed behind to write about owning one's body through herbal remedies for everything from headache to schizophrenia, and we are on the move. Here's the red VW, dented and dirty, puffs of smoke from its exhaust, tilted like it can barely stay on the road, six kids inside, our faces pushed up against the glass. Jacob does the Dr. Strangelove getting-strangled-by-your-own-hand gag, his tongue sticking out. Micah and I watch for big rigs, we make the pull-the-horn gesture and go crazy with joy when the trucker toots his horn for us.

We've been on the road for three days.

Dad plays a tape of *Mystery Theater* and I listen to the long, drawn-out sound of the squeaky door at the opening of the episode. I chew on a pillow in my nest, listening. The episode is almost over, my heart going fast in my chest, and then a horrible, wet sound effect.

Oh. Oh. My. God, says a character. He's—he's *inside out*!!

Own your own body, turn yourself inside out like a sock, organs pulsing, serpentine intestines wet and alive. Mom wrote a poem, *I turn my heart inside out / and wear it that way for you*. My own heart cranks up, I am shaking on my pile of blankets and suitcases, my insides at risk of terrifying exposure.

It's moonless black when we get to the farmhouse. Fireflies blink between trees. We pile out of the VW, road stink released into breathing forest. It was once a blueberry farm, now the bushes have gone tall and wild.

In the morning, Dad goes to DC for a conference. On the kitchen counter he leaves two bags of groceries to last the week, or maybe two weeks, that he'll be gone.

That night we roast hot dogs over a fire in the pit down the slope. Marshmallows bubble black and crisp on the outside, gloriously sticky inside.

Day two. The grocery bags on the kitchen counter are empty, one lying on its side like a lost sock.

Leda stomps to the porch.

Who ate all the *food*? she yells.

My brothers look blankly in her direction. We don't have an answer. The food was there and we ate it.

Leda is eighteen and meant to be our stand-in mom, but she has no authority. We're stuck here at the farm, thirty miles from the nearest town. The only car is the old Falcon in the barn, and it can barely manage to rumble to the end of the dirt road and back.

We'll have to make do, says Leda, using Dad's phrase.

There are blueberries ripe on the bushes, and flour, salt, shortening, and sugar in the pantry. We're used to slim rations at the end of most months when the money runs out, cooked cabbage and powdered milk. We know how to make do.

Micah and I go out with big tin cans to gather blueberries. Our cans are heaped high so fast we catch the overflow in our T-shirts, waddle back awkwardly with can held close to chest, T-shirt hem in the other hand, blueberries spilling out the sides. Leda and I make two blueberry pies for dinner. We discipline ourselves: just one pie eaten, the other saved for tomorrow.

Day three. I'm awake early. I stand in the kitchen looking at the pie, smooth lid of crust. Just one piece. I slice into the pie and a spurt of ants rushes up and over the crust. It's only a few, I can brush them away and still save the pie, but when I pull out the piece the whole inside is alive with ants. Nightmare creatures crawling over each other on jittery legs, black and shining. I clatter the knife to the counter and jump back, unable to unstick my eyes from the horror.

Day four. In the forest, Micah catches an eft and I a toad. We carry them back to the farmhouse in our hands as we discuss licking the toad, both of us sharing a hazy idea of hallucinations from licking toads or maybe frogs. Neither of us can remember which. The older brothers admire our catch.

It's toads that are hallucinogenic, says Jacob.

Dare you, says Luke.

I stick out my tongue a millimeter from the toad's breathing back, closer, closer, touch the tip to its flesh. I giggle, breathless with my daring, but the boys are already gone, heading for the rope swing. I let the toad go, squat to watch him gulp and blink. He pops into a sudden leap and crashes down, leap, crash.

Day five. Blueberry pancakes made with canned milk. We forget to bathe. We are alive with hunger, my hipbones sharp in my too-small red-white-and-blue shorts. We've gone feral, barefoot and tangle-haired in the Pennsylvania forest.

I'm in the kitchen with a comic book. I lean casually against the stove, trying to look grown-up. I rest my arm on the stove. It feels ice-cold then hot, and when I yank my arm back it sticks then peels.

Wait, I think. I take it back, I think.

Then the pain rushes in and I slide to the floor, open my mouth to wail. My loud *waaaah waaaah waaaah*. I let loose and then stop for a breath. I'm curious. Hiccupping and sniffling, I bend my arm up with the other hand so I can see the long curve darkening red. Leda finds me here and we put my arm under cold water until it numbs, my whole arm spanking red. I will have the scar for years. It will teach me right from left; all I have to do is look at the inside of my forearm, the left one with its sickle burn.

We don't know what else to do for the burn. I insist on a bandage and we find gauze in the bathroom cabinet. It will stick to the burn and peel it weeping raw all over again when I take it off.

Day six. Brothers roll the Falcon out of the barn. Leda watches from the porch. She isn't sure we should but she has no energy to argue. The brothers take turns behind the wheel, driving it slow down Myers road and back. Micah and I beg.

Me too, me too, we say.

Luke gets out of the car and bows, holding the door open. Micah slides in behind the wheel and I'm next to him. He's too short to reach the pedals, so he steers while I crouch on the floorboard, press the gas, the brake.

Go, says Micah. Slower. Stop, stop!

We're at the end of the road. Jonah hops in and turns the car around. This time I get to steer. I'm stretching up as far as I can to see over the long hood.

Goooo, I say. Wait, wait!

The steering wheel is sliding through my hands and I panic. I forget to tell Micah to stop and the car veers wild to the right. I overcorrect and see sky, trees—I let go a yell as we dive into the ditch. We sit stunned. I have the sick feeling I'm about to get into big trouble. We have to crawl out the passenger side.

Dummy! yell the brothers. What'd you *do*?

Leda and I watch while the boys push the Falcon up and out of the ditch. They walk around the car, slide hands over the bumper and doors feeling for damage. Leda lets a breath out through her teeth and Jonah looks up, shrugs one shoulder. They roll it back into the barn, close the door behind it.

My bandage is already filthy, the end hanging loose and frayed. I tuck it under the rest of the bandage, tuck it again, tuck it again.

Day seven. Sick of blueberries. I'm carrying a full tin back to the farmhouse and stuff my cheeks. I start to chew but it's too much, I open my mouth and let a clump fall into the undergrowth. My stomach grinds.

Rain. Straight fat drops splat leaves all around the farmhouse. Rain sizzles on the porch. I run outside and dance in it, T-shirt and shorts wetted to my body, bandage sopped. I put my head back and open my mouth to let rain fall in, fill me up, my arms open, elbows hyperextended like birdwings. I'm a goshdarn prima ballerina, I'm Titania, I'm queen of the forest. I dance until my breath runs out and then I stand, face up to the sky, watch raindrops drilling down down, keep my eyes open in the swim as long as I can.

Day we've-lost-track. Dad returns. He is back and we eat as though we will never eat again because now we know. We know anything can happen.

The folding door at the back of the Relief Society room is open to show the baptismal font, blue swimming pool water, Celestial chlorine clean. Mormons are baptized at the age of eight. Baptism on Saturday, and then on Sunday I'll be confirmed, a full member of the Church.

My father in white holds his hand high behind my head while he recites the baptismal prayer. The water is up to my ribs. I bend my knees and he lays me backward in the water while I hold my nose, then he pulls me up again against all that water. I'm getting ready to climb out, but there's a quiet commotion among the men in their black suits. It seems the end of my braid floated up; I wasn't completely immersed. A mite of sin holding to the tip of my braid. They call for a do-over. Dad does the prayer again and grabs my braid and dunks me with gusto so I lose grip on my nose and one foot floats up, cold air on my toe. It feels sloppy, but they call it good. We slosh our way up and out of the font.

I'm not sure I believe in my cleanliness. That toe poking out of the water, like Achilles's heel. I want to get back in, try and try until we get it right.

I want to believe I can be good from now on.

But I won't. I'll sin again. Within the hour I'll pick a fight with my brother.

I will sin again with my cousin.

In years to come I will sin a million times.

There's a picture from this day, of Mom and me. I'm in my white baptismal dress and white bow, and Mom is crouched behind me, gripping my shoulders while I have a stranglehold on our calico kitten, Rover Cleveland.

Mom looks happy. She's slim, hair in a Dorothy Hamill cut. I'm grinning toothlessly into the camera, sinless for a minute.

In the cupboard of cleaning supplies is a bottle of furniture polish. It is golden yellow. When I open the cupboard, sun through the open door lights it up. I have been thinking about it for a while now, opening the cupboard to look, closing it again. My best friend is lost to me, safe in the Celestial Kingdom. She died before anything she did counted as a sin, because Heavenly Father knew she was better than me, because she didn't have to be tested. I want to blink out, like she did. I want a funeral and friends crying about me, snot running down their faces. Before the furniture polish, I experimented with nasal spray, tried spraying it in my mouth instead of my nose. I half-knew it wouldn't do anything but tried it anyway, putting the medicine where it wasn't supposed to go. The furniture polish, however, has clear warnings on the label. I lift the bottle to drink. Maybe I only want to get sick. Maybe I only want attention. Maybe a will to live, guilt over the sin of suicide keeps me from drinking more than a few swallows.

My stomach rejects the furniture polish. I am vomiting, but this is nothing new. Nobody knows what I did.

Dad opens Leda's bedroom door late on Christmas Eve, movie camera running. Leda's in there, fluffs of batten in her hair and stuck to her turtleneck, her hands feeding fabric into the sewing machine. It's after midnight, she's almost nineteen, and her eyes glint bright black. She's been working for weeks to make stuffed sea monsters for the brothers, six feet long in hallucinatory colors.

After Dad goes to sleep, Leda creeps out to the Christmas tree to arrange her creations. On the fireplace is a heavy wooden box. She opens it to see a full set of secondhand silverware, floral sculpted handles. For her hope chest, she's sure of it. She gave her childhood over to raising us, now it's her turn.

Christmas morning. I'm the first one up. Dad has placed one of his big paintings across the entrance to the living room. I have to roust everyone from bed, lead Dad by the hand to move the painting for the big reveal.

There are no wrapped presents, just Leda's sea monsters. A doll she made for me. The box of silverware.

Leda's face goes marble. Smooth and perfect as a cameo. The silverware is a gift from Dad to Mom. Leda will not allow anyone to see her cry. Dad points the camera at her. She stares death rays straight into the lens. He moves on to my brothers. Jonah, Luke, Jacob, every one glares flat into the camera's eye, the camera Dad's shield. Even Micah looks up as Dad calls his name, then away and down, shaking his blond sleep-rubbed head. They're all years too old for sea monsters, for sea monsters and nothing, nothing else.

Is it really true, I'll ask my sister when we're grown. Were there really no presents?

Nothing at all, she'll say.

In the home movie, I dance the doll Leda made in front of the camera. My pretend child, long brown braids like my own.

It is 1978, and Dad is directing a study abroad in Paris, the whole mob of us fresh from Utah in France for an entire semester. We climb out of the bus from the airport with our suitcases, drag them behind us up the narrow street to our apartment. An apartment! There is a tiny balcony, a gesture toward one anyway, an inch of concrete bounded by a railing. I lean out over the railing. Down at street level is a pair of humping dogs. Across the alley, another apartment building—I look for an uncurtained window, a glimpse of other lives.

Mom and Dad get the master bedroom. The four boys are stacked in bunkbeds in the second room. Leda and I get bunkbeds in the living room. We shift the bookshelf to partition our area from the rest of the room, an idea of privacy. I've gotten permission to finish fourth grade via home study, and I stack my textbooks on the shelf. I will put off homework as long as I can, finishing the whole school year in the last week before it's due.

Mom retreats to the bedroom, and Leda and Dad go out to find food. They come back with their arms full, long loaves laid onto the small round dinner table.

These, says Dad, his mouth just holding back a laugh, are *baguettes*.

Do they have giant ones called *bags*? says Jacob.

No no, says Luke. It's like a tiny wife. I'd like to introduce you to the old bagu*ette*.

We sit around the table, jet-lagged, dazzled with newness, laughing ourselves silly.

The students live in a *pension* in another part of the city. We have dinners there with the students, and classes are also held there. The students become my social circle, never mind I'm ten years younger than them: my Paris life is bigger, brighter, more grown-up than my Provo life could ever be.

I have a shiny black map of the Paris Metro. The lines are marked out in candy-bright colors. Dad gets me a *Carte Orange*, a laminated Metro pass with my big dumb Utah face shining out. He shows us the way from home to the pension and back.

To get home, explains Dad, you go toward Mairie d'Issy.

Think of it as *Marie is here*, he says, So you want to go toward Mom. And then our stop is Volontaires, because you volunteer to go there.

Orientation is complete. Dad goes to teach, Mom finds her spot in bed, and we kids are loosed on the city. In Provo I'm limited to where I can ride a bike and have to tackle the long steep climb home. Here, at nine years old, I can explore the city alone. Paris is mine.

The Metro map is beautiful. It has a newness about it, a clarity. Those bright colors translate to real places. Pasteur station is shining pink tiles, and Louis Pasteur's penicillin will forever be pink in my imagination.

Joanie is braiding my hair. We're in the room she shares with three other BYU students.

Don't go out alone after dark, says Joanie.

Carlos the Jackal is here, you know, says Michelle.

I don't know who he is, but his name pops in my mouth like firecrackers. *Carlos the Jackal.*

You have to watch out for white slavers, says Joanie. She nods her head with import.

I get stuck on this, like a record with a skip. *White slavers.* Do they wear white? Are they white? I picture men with pure white hair and bubble sunglasses like Andy Warhol. I picture white sails on a pirate ship. The modifier makes it more mysterious and almost glamorous.

It will be some time before I realize it's because the slavers want white girls, and it will be longer before I become conscious of the violence in this expression, in separating *slavers* from *white slavers*, in assigning greater horror to the idea of slavery when the victims are white-skinned.

The students tell me not to go out alone after dark, but I stay late at the pension with my new friends. Sunset is early; we've arrived in Paris in midwinter. Many evenings I crunch home through snow long after dark, the streets quiet and the sound of my own footsteps echo like someone behind me, some monster, matching my stride. I count my steps and my toes go numb in the sharp cold and my pulse pounds in my ears, I am scared, but the fear wakes me, moves me. I grow larger and stranger out here in the dark.

At the pension is a long curving staircase with a faded floral rug. Jonah does fake falls down these stairs. He's tall, he throws his body down the stairs with maximum ruckus, lets his arms and legs hit loud and reverberate, he punctuates his fall with exclamations, *Ow! Hey! Wha—?* until he comes to rest at last at the bottom.

Do it again! I say, clapping. Do it again!

He laughs and hops to his feet, and then he's out the door and gone in the streets of Paris.

Many years later, when I'm grown, Leda will tell me she fell down those stairs for real. At the bottom, she was knocked unconscious. I was with her. She'll tell me I got her home, that she doesn't remember the journey, only that she came to herself again at our apartment.

Our parents know nothing of Leda's fall. When we are grown, we will sit at the dinner table and fill our parents with the stories they never knew.

I don't want to hear it, Mom will say. If I didn't know then, I don't want to know now.

Why didn't you tell us? Dad will say.

We will laugh. We are heartless. Mom will put her hands over her ears.

Do you remember, we'll say, when Jacob stole the car and passed Dad on the road and he never saw him?

Totally oblivious!

You know I sneaked out my bedroom every night?

Mom will leave the table, disappear into the bedroom.

Every night? No way.

Every night.

Remember when Luke was threatened at knifepoint?

And then he made friends with the muggers!

You sneaked out every night, really?

Back in Provo, I would be sitting in my fourth-grade classroom right now. Mr. Anderson teaching metric conversions. Instead I'm in Luxembourg Gardens. An old Frenchman in aviator sunglasses shows me how to play boules. He puts the ball in my hand and pantomimes the throw. I loft the ball wildly, it drops and scatters a mess of pigeons. Wings flash large, bird bodies lift, tucking up their claws.

I can sit in on BYU classes if I like. Ancient flowered wallpaper is on the classroom walls, windows along one side to the street below. I decide which classes are interesting: French, History (sometimes), Art (Dad's class). But I don't have to show up at all.

In Provo, Stacy or Lisa or Jennifer would call me Greaseball in the hallway. Here I'm anonymous and dorky in braids and overalls. A French girl on the Metro with her mother wears straight-leg jeans and a big cashmere sweater, hair curling down her back. Her expression says that I'm beneath her notice and I can't even take it personally. It's just how it is.

You're a hundred times more sophisticated than me, I think. But you're holding your Mommy's hand and I'm alone. I can do anything I like.

Mom crochets in Paris. She makes delicate white rosettes with the tiniest of crochet hooks.

I don't know what I'm making, Mom announces.

The rosettes multiply.

Leda and I walk to the Metro from the pension one night. It's raining. I see a man running, water splashes up from his feet, his pant legs speckled dark. Daylight is gone. Leda stops and takes my hand. The man slows to long steps, and we see where he is pointed. Parisians begin to clot the space, their black umbrellas closing in. At their feet is a figure in the gutter. I see a delicate white wrist. I see red foaming in the gutter stream. Two gendarmes flank an old man with a large basset hound face. His profile glows against dark rain. His big sad Gallic nose. His hands are held awkwardly in front of his ribs, and I understand that he is cuffed.

Leda will remember a single lighted balcony above, a person silhouetted in the light, looking down.

I don't know if I see the knife. I don't know if I hear the French word for *stab*, but I know that is what happened. Leda and I remain at a distance. We do not join the crowd. We stand in the rain for I don't know how long and then Leda pulls me away. I glimpse the body again as we pass: a woman. This is what happens when a woman dares to be alone. She is unprotected, a soft target, her body open to the knife.

Leda keeps hold of my hand as we walk on, as we descend stately on the escalator into the deeps of the Metro. In the train, she puts an arm around my shoulders.

~

I'm late getting home. I was up too long with the students and it's well past any acceptable hour. I'm alone on a nearly empty metro car. A tall woman slouches in the seat facing mine, legs stretched in front of her, confident as a man. She is so grave I doubt myself: woman or man? She stares me down, white-faced, eyes flat, unreadable. I can't look away. I think about white slavers, about Carlos the Jackal, about murderers. At my stop I jump out, heart pounding in my ears. I run up the stairs and out of the metro station, run all the way to our apartment building, do not dare to look over my shoulder. I'll be killed by the woman or by Dad for staying out late. The elevator in our building is broken so it's a dash all the way up, five floors, I'm panting. At the door, I gulp my breath, open the door as slow as I can manage. Maybe I can creep in and only Leda will know, everyone else asleep in their rooms.

All the lights in the apartment are on.

That's it, I think. I'm dead.

The whole family is crowded around the too-small dining table. I slip in unnoticed. My brother has had an accident.

Wanna see? says Jonah.

We all lean in. He stretches out his wrist to show. It is sewn together with big shiny stitches, thick black knots along the top like spines on a dinosaur's back. I don't understand why it doesn't have a white bandage, why they leave it all hanging out in the open like that. Those big shining loops look sloppy to me, like the doctors rushed their work. As of this moment, I disapprove of French doctors.

Fell down the stairs in the Metro, he says.

I picture him falling comically, loudly down the stairs in the pension. What station? I think. I try to picture very sharp stairs, gray concrete with blades of steel at the corners. How do you cut your wrist falling down stairs? I think.

He was carrying a bottle of Coke, says Dad, as if he hears my thoughts. It broke.

A few bottles, says Jonah.

One day I will understand it was no accident. The creature in Mom's brain passed down, come to life in my generation.

~

Micah and I are peeling potatoes. We stand together at the sink, and he puts a finger to his lips, eyes smiling at me. He drops the peeler with a clatter, grabs at his wrist, runs howling to the WC and turns on the water. Mom stands close to me in the kitchen. It's a small kitchen. I see all the muscles in her face let go at once. Her skin sags like a dampened handkerchief.

No, she says. Almost to herself.

She's still for half a second, then twitches into motion, runs after him.

Micah's crouched over the sink, pretending to sob. He turns as Mom closes him in her arms, and now she sees there's no blood, he's laughing, his blond hair against her chest.

Ah. Mom lets air go out of her body with a fast breath. Ah. I see tears held in her eyes by a single molecule layer of tension.

Don't do that, she says. Her voice isn't scolding. She pleads with him.

Please, she says. Don't do that. Ever again.

Micah's laugh stops and his arms go around her.

I'm sorry, Mom. I'm sorry, he says.

We are all of us standing in the kitchen, frozen in mid-dinner prep. Leda with a kitchen towel in one hand. Water boiling on the stove. We watch Mom and Micah with their arms around each other.

Mom in Paris is Skinny, her Calvin Klein jeans zipped all the way, a white bandage patch over one eye. None of my siblings will remember why she wore a patch.

An infection? Leda will say.

We do not know. But she wears this patch and her smile pops, as though she has successfully pushed her hell into a single eye and caught the poison in the white bandage on her face, loosening her body, opening her up. I see her toss her hair back and smile over one shoulder at Dad.

In Provo, violence moves in a slow rot beneath the surface, hidden under bright Utah smiles. Here in Paris it crackles along the top. Here it splits open your day and there are no secrets, no shame. We hang beside each other and move in reverential slowness around the shattered front of a café beside the pension, turned inside out by a firebomb. I vibrate with this surface ferocity. Paris feels like a home, home for the smarter, sharper version of me.

Here I'm freer than I've ever been. With dinners at the pension and a small apartment, housework is minimal. I don't have to go to school. My kid brain picks up French, and Micah and I approach fluency. We do the shopping for the whole family. I imagine myself living here, in a garret by the Seine, and for once my fantasy does not end with a wedding. The story is mine alone.

We've been abroad for six months, returning now to the US. The plane tilts into a landing at the Salt Lake airport. It's June and there is still snow on the peaks of the mountains. My heart jumps. Is my home really so beautiful? Outside, I breathe in sharp, dry Utah air. I didn't know I'd missed it so much.

In August, Leda marries the man she'd been writing to from Paris, her own happy-ever-aftering. I am a flower girl with Chrissie's sister, Betsy—my new best friend, my cruelty forgiven or just left aside, both of us trying to fill the hole Chrissie left in our lives—in brown dresses. Like my sister and new brother-in-law, Betsy and I had sent each other long letters on blue airmail paper, her round handwriting better than mine will ever be. Mom's endless white rosettes become the bodice of my sister's dress, Mom nodding at her own clairvoyance.

In Provo, the Fourth of July is celebrated all day, ending with an orgy of fireworks spread across the sky. With funding from the Osmond family, we get the biggest fireworks display in the whole United States. From our house on the side of the mountain, with our giant windows, we have front-row seats. The show is synced with music from the classical station on the radio, and it builds in a slow crescendo, ending with twenty rockets launched at once in a massive, thundering climax.

Here, today, in the Springville Art Museum is Leda's happy ending, her exploding fireworks, her debut as a full woman, a Mrs.—she has taken on her husband's name like a queen's ermine robe. Leda's wedded to a man with a cop mustache in a tan tux, who will go on to become a prison guard, then warden of the state penitentiary. Leda will break free of our home and shut herself up in one of her own, and I am delirious with the fantasy of the day. I love being her flower girl, love the tall baskets of sunflowers at the reception, the pastel candied almonds, the circlet of white blossoms around my sister's head. And then the wedding is over and she's gone.

I didn't count on this. She's just gone. I'm left alone with my savage brothers in our house wedged into the side of the mountain.

The Aughts

I'M BLEEDING, STILL. I'VE STARTED talking about my pads and tampons as my dressing, as in a wound dressing, as in I have to change my dressing. I duck into the bathroom at the mortuary to change my dressing. I'm thin from months of bleeding and no appetite, wrists poking out from my sleeves like I've gotten too tall for my shirts. Hair prickly, growing out after I shaved it down, streamlining myself. If my family is hyperreal, I feel myself receding from the corporeal world, pedaling backward somewhere along the trail Mom left behind. A nurse said I was close to death the night Gabe brought me in for a transfusion, and I was okay with that—a painless enough fadeout, first me then Mom.

Dad asks me to speak at the funeral. My bloodstarved brain spins.

Sunday. The family goes to church. I tell them I don't feel up to it, and lie with my husband in the basement room that was mine when I was in college. We have tender, bloody, guilty sex.

The funeral is on Monday. I wear the dark plum dress I'd picked out for Grandma and Grandpa's funeral. Now officially my funeral dress. The viewing first: Mom in her white temple clothes. There's a bonnet on the pillow above her head. Before they close the casket, the mortician starts to put the bonnet on Mom's head. My sister is standing beside me holding my hand, but at this she moves fast to the casket. She pushes the mortician aside and adjusts the bonnet, ties it under Mom's chin in a bow. Is this what they wear in the temple? It looks ridiculous, a lunch lady hat with a bow under the chin.

One by one, my brothers and my father move to her side, all of them now at the casket. I do not follow. I stay where I am. Stubborn. I don't know why. I don't know what principle I'm defending. I'm not repulsed, it's nothing like that. Only that isn't Mom. It's just skin in the shape of her. The rubber-mask mouth set in disappointment. My mother no longer exists.

Or, worse: she exists, but inanimate, uncomprehending, a pile of meat that once breathed and thought of itself as an *I*, a human with meaning and purpose. And now the machine has broken down, it doesn't mean anything anymore.

In the entrance to the sacrament room at church is one of Dad's paintings of Mom, Mom full-length and life-size and graceful in a towel, her neck long. Slightly scandalous to show such a thing in the church, but we're allowed some leeway in our grief. It fits us, fits Mom's flamboyance. My turn to speak. I get up and read one of her poems, sit down again. After the funeral Dad puts on his coachman's hat and tails, climbs up front with the coachman for the Black Mariah, and we creep behind them all the way to the cemetery on the far side of town.

At the graveside, Dad is talking with his old friend Edie, their heads leaning toward each other. Edie and her husband Jim were my parents' best friends. They are divorced now; Jim was arrested years ago for fraud. Leda and I look at them and Leda gives me a private smile. After the funeral we're counting up casseroles from the neighborhood widows. Dad won't be single long. He's made for love. Dad is as much a flirt as Mom ever was, as much as I am.

1980

MOM HAS PROMISED THAT WHEN I am twelve I can wear my hair in a French twist. I'm doing my own hair now, spend an hour getting it right on the Sunday after my birthday. I carry my head differently at church, officially a young woman. At school I'm in orchestra (violin), band (clarinet), and guitar class. I inherited my siblings' outgrown musical instruments, carry them all with me to school—two instruments in one hand, one in the other, book bag over my shoulder, a nerd in full flower. After school is ballet, then *Coppélia* rehearsals, hours of ballet every night. I want to do all of it, hungry for the world; I am not growing up fast enough, my body not wide enough to hold everything I want to be.

Mom loans me a mystery novel.

This book is so good, she says. You'll love it!

Mom reading mysteries means she's near full power. At her best, she reads poetry and literature. Mysteries when her mind wants a little break. From there on down through levels of depression: Harlequin romances, *Vogue* magazine, nothing at all.

She and I both cling to reading like a life raft. I tear through books, eating words as fast as I can. I've already pulled *Ulysses* from the shelf, already my brothers snorted with laughter when I asked the meaning of *scrotum-tightening* at the dinner table. (Leda clued me in a week later, explaining through blushes and not-quite-suppressed hilarity the effect of cold on a man's anatomy.)

So I tuck happily into the thick book Mom handed me, a recommendation from Mom, rare and precious. It's a decent story, pulls me along; though it ain't literature, it's okay for a Saturday read.

And then the sex scene. *Ulysses* was impenetrable enough that I didn't quite pick up on its crassness, but this book is precise, near clinical in its descriptions. A long page goes into embroidered detail of cunnilingus: the protagonist pulling back at the very moment the woman begins to move her hips, he cruelly leaves her hanging.

I realize my mouth is open, drying out. People *do* that? I think. And then: *Mom* read this! Finally: *Mom gave it to me*. I can't make it hang right in my head.

Mom, I say. Why did you give me this?

What? she says. Didn't you like it?

Mom, I say. Mom. The sex!

Sex . . . ?

Mom, there's a whole long sex scene! And more than that. But this one, it's . . . Mom, it's explicit.

Mom looks at me for half a second, then lets go a laugh.

Oh honey, she shakes her head. I completely forgot about that.

I am doubtful. To me those words stand out in a blaze. Who cares who the killer was? A man licked a woman's private parts. Clearly Mom didn't remember this part because she's innocent in a way I will never be, her mind skipped right by. I am all the way wrong. I got excited, then embarrassed at the description of the woman's response, her moving hips, shameful enough to make him stop. Okay, I think. It's better to just hold still. Don't let on that you like it.

When I get my first zit, I'm stoked. Years of long evenings lounging on the bed with the TV on, Mom popping zits on my brothers' backs, I've finally caught up. Luke tries to tell me how to pop it, but I'm not quite following.

Here, he says. He picks up a shard of soap and draws a zit on the bathroom mirror, arrows pointing to the base of the zit at the angle I should employ. We leave this zit diagram on the bathroom mirror for weeks, and more weeks, until the soap flakes away, but still the ghost of the picture appears when the mirror fogs over.

The feeling of belonging doesn't last. I get a sudden rush of zits and cysts and boils across my face, crowding each other, fighting for space on my skin. Nothing on my back for Mom to pop, and I'm impatient, I dig at the cysts until my face is bleeding. I'm sent to the dermatologist, a friend of the family who writes me a prescription for tetracycline, and then erythromycin two years later. The drugs only just keep my acne this side of horrific.

Look at you, says Mom. You're almost a teenager and you have all these hormones running around your body.

In Mom's southern Utah accent, it's *harmones*.

My body has harmones running around it and Mom writes *poims*.

I correct her, like the snotty preteen I am.

It's HOR-mones, Mom. PO-em, I say.

Now she looks at me uncertainly when she speaks.

Hooooormones, she says, reverting to her tentative self. *Po-em*.

Mom brings me a sheaf of her poetry.

Read these for me, she says. Tell me what you think.

Be brutal, she says.

Apparently she thinks I'm old enough now, suddenly my opinion matters. The task is impossible. I have to read them at an agonized slant: love poems for Dad, poems about depression, poems about sex. If I really am brutal, I could drive her right back into bed. I keep them for a week, then hand them back with vague words of praise. I can't do anything else.

The creative energy that drives you to make art, says Mom, is the same as the impulse to make babies.

She spent all that creative energy on us. It's our fault she hasn't done more with her poetry. She is so insecure in her own work that she gives it to me to critique, and this is my fault too.

~

When I get my period, Dad is the one to buy my pads. At Family Home Drag, Jacob stands up to announce that I need to Do Something about my used pads. I've been keeping them in a brown paper bag that I carry into my room, but one day I forgot and left it on the back of the toilet.

I saw the bag, says Jacob, and thought it might be something good. Like a sandwich? And then I looked inside and almost threw up! Like, disgusting bloody pads!

I've traumatized my brother, shamed myself forever. Okay then. Never again. (But it isn't never. I leave a bloodstain on the sheet when I'm a houseguest and am too ashamed to mention it. My periods are heavy and irregular and last too long, I'm caught unprepared almost every time—I leak, I ruin my clothes, targets of blood on the backs of my skirts, concentric rings moving outward in lighter and lighter brownish reds.)

Twenty-five years from now, I will break down in the shower. I will fold myself into a corner of the tub, water hitting my naked body. I will never have a period again.

Unwoman, I will think. I'm not a woman anymore.

In one corner of the living room is one of Dad's biggest kinetic light sculptures. He collaborates with his brother Bob, the electrical engineer. This one is called Pillar of Light, and it's a representation of Joseph Smith's vision, where Heavenly Father and Jesus Christ appeared in a pillar of light descending from heaven.

Our living room has ten-foot ceilings. Pillar of Light reaches almost exactly floor to ceiling. It is a column of white Plexiglas. If you could look at it from above, it would be shaped like an eye. When you plug it in, it lights up inside. A bright sunny yellow at the top, it cascades into oranges and reds and pinks and whites in a column all the way down to the floor. The lights dim and brighten and subtly shift in color. There is no base to the sculpture. Plexiglas just meets carpet.

I am vacuuming. I put off vacuuming as long as I can, but once I begin I get absorbed in the task. Vacuuming is satisfying. I try to make even stripes in the carpet. When Leda got married we recarpeted, a burnt orangey red with a sheen to it. I make one golden-red stripe by pulling the vacuum backward against the nap, one silky dark stripe by pushing it forward. Light stripe, dark stripe. Light stripe, dark stripe. I come close to the base of the sculpture but quickly pull the vacuum back while angling it into a new stripe. Close and then back. On my last pass, I bump the vacuum against the bottom of the sculpture.

Tink.

The vacuum makes that sound as it hits the sculpture. It's not loud. Tink.

And the Pillar of Light falls.

It is a terrible long instant. I jump back and pull the vacuum out of its path. For an age I watch it tip, and nothing to be done. The thing outweighs me. This blank, clean white Plexiglas face hides guts of electronic hardware, bulbs and sockets and wires and Uncle Bob's solid-state circuitry. It falls graceful as an archangel.

And then it bounces. The side that was the back is now the top, shattering. Thick white Plexiglas breaks along curving, sinuous lines. I can hear bulbs pop, Bang, Bang, Bang. And then it's quiet.

I do not know what happens next. My memory sticks and judders here, the ruined giant at my feet. I must tell Dad, but I have cleared this moment from my tapes. I don't know if Dad says it outright, or if we just silently agree it would be best if I stay out of his way for a while. Either way, I manage to be out of the room whenever Dad is around. I get my own breakfast early, before anyone else is up. I eat dinner late, after everyone else is done. If nothing is left, I steam myself some broccoli. We steer clear of each other for about two weeks, and then we never speak of it again.

It's night. I'm alone, reading on the love seat Dad hammered together from scraps of wood. Mom emerges from her room at the end of the hallway, sits next to me in the darkened living room.

I'm looking out over the city from our giant windows. Mom looks at the wall.

Have you ever been . . . molested, by one of your relatives? she says.

My heart grips hard inside me. The memory emerges against my will, pulled up like a rabbit out of a hat. I want to lean into her. Mom, I want to say, You see it. You see me.

Yes, I say.

She seems to draw into herself. She is looking down at the space between us on the love seat.

Who was—she begins. She corrects herself. I don't need to know, she says. Just tell me he's been through the temple.

He has, I say.

Good, she says. She nods to the space between our hands. That means he's reconciled with Heavenly Father.

She gets up and goes to her room.

I'm left in the dark, the city lit up below.

Maybe, I think, it never happened after all.

Otherwise she would have taken me in her arms.

Mormons believe that, after a righteous life, you can become a god in the next life. This is the whole point. You come to earth, get a body, die, become a god, and populate your own worlds with spirit children.

To achieve this, you must be married. Unmarried people, however righteous, will never ascend higher than ministering angels.

Gods and goddesses. Not just peace. Not just mansions in heaven. The most grandiose of ambitions answered: to become a god.

Mom has been well enough long enough to have a job. With the extra money, Dad buys her a car, a Mercury Bobcat. He thinks it's a sports car. My brothers are all car guys; Dad, not so much. He thinks he's given Mom a splendid gift.

Mom hates it. She drives it only a handful of times and it reverts to Dad, then me when I get my driver's license. Years later, she will finally have a real sports car, a red RX-7. For now, she poses for Dad who snaps a photo. Mom in a yellow dress, leaning against her yellow Bobcat.

Mom lifts her chin like a 1940s fashion model. This is her photo pose, her mirror pose: chin up, hair tossed back.

Near the end of her life, that chin lift will look like she is trying not to drown.

Second wiving.

Wife: twelve-year-old girl.

Husband: redhaired Dan from across town. He is fifteen and I met him at a friend's house. He calls to ask me to go running with him.

Yes, I say. Of course. Of course I'll go running.

I meet him at the park and it's evening. It's getting dark when we get to a chapel on the far edge of town. We're on the long lawn of the church when he leans in close. I am looking at his mouth, his wet red lips, and then he's kissing me. My first kiss.

My head is cranked back to kiss him, and then he hugs me to his chest, velour shirt, my nose full of his deodorant. It's dark now and he starts to talk. He's holding me close and he's warning me about slow dancing with boys.

And then he sticks his tongue in my ear. It crackles loudly.

A sweet shock rolls down my body. My ear is wet. I smell saliva.

This is the devil, he whispers.

He's so serious. I want to laugh. But it is the devil and I've stopped resisting.

We are walking up the long hill to my house when Dad drives by in the VW bus. Dad has a special facility for not noticing. I will walk right by him on BYU campus and he will never see me, no jolt of recognition, nothing. But tonight of all nights, in the dark, he sees me walking home with Dan. I give him a complicated, implausible story about my friend Elizabeth, how she was with us but she had a night class at BYU. I repeat the story to Mom, the smell of Dan's deodorant still with me. Mom's face dulls into disappointment. She won't say she knows I'm lying but I can see it.

Third wiving.

Wife: sixth grader, last year of elementary school.

Husband: Robert Fagg, the paperboy.

Robert Fagg stands on a wooden stool below my bedroom window, thrums his fingertips on the glass. It's five a.m. and I'm still in my nightgown. I stand on my bed and open the window for him.

He's fifteen and I'm twelve and he is all delicious bad boy. In the neighborhood someone yells *Fagg* down the street and Robert turns, lifts a chin to challenge anyone who would mess with him.

Yeah? he says.

I lean out my window to kiss him, let him (sin sin sin) feel my breasts.

BYU campus is my second living room. When I was little Dad took me here, and while he taught I ran wild in the halls of the Harris Fine Arts Center. There was an ice cream vending machine in the basement, and Dad's colleague, Mr. Burnside, who was a thousand years old and never married, held my hand and asked me serious questions and bought me ice cream sandwiches. I sat on his desk and swung my feet and we talked about art and stars and how to grow vegetables and ballet. I ate ice cream sandwiches and this is how it is supposed to be, old man and little girl. We could talk because we both had time.

Mr. Burnside retired and I got older and time ran through my hands, and now I'm twelve and the Harris Fine Arts Center is too small for me. I wander farther and today I'm at the student union. The cafeteria is on the ground floor, and upstairs are couches and pictures of BYU beauty queens, and on the mezzanine is a piano.

Fourth wiving.

Wife: still twelve. Not yet in junior high.

Husband: the pianist has long, feathered blond hair, illegally long for a man on BYU campus. He smiles at me over the keys. I lean against the piano and watch him play. I'm wearing rope-soled sandals that feel glamorous.

I am flirting. He looks up at me, his blue eyes focus on mine. He tells me his name is Dave H. His crutches rest against the piano.

He likes me, I think. It's a revelation.

I tell him I have to go home, I've left my things in a cloakroom upstairs. He gets up from the piano and follows me to the elevator on crutches. One foot is bandaged. I am magic, this man is following me. I imagine kissing, tipping my face up and his arms around me.

We're in the elevator and he stands close to me. He is twenty-six years old. He smiles down at me and his front tooth is broken. My body flushes all over with sick fascination. I want him, I don't want him in the elevator with me.

I am not at all sure of myself, not in the way that is necessary now.

We get to the sixth floor and I stick in place. He stands in the door of the elevator, the doors bumping against him, and holds his hand out to coax me.

I step out of the elevator.

Oh, *I* know this place, he says. And he's off on his crutches, he finds my coat and bag, hanging all by themselves on the empty rack. I catch up to him, reach for my coat. He smells like cigarettes, like Uncle Stan, like the Paris Metro. Tobacco is a sin but I love its evil man-smell.

His crutches clatter to the floor behind him and he leans into me. I stumble under his weight, I fold. My bottom hits floor, we are an awkward mess of arms and legs.

He doesn't kiss me. His hand is undoing my pants and I feel air on bare skin. I gulp in a breath.

Don't scream, he says.

I hadn't thought of screaming. My voice has gone missing from my throat.

He is giving me instructions like a teacher. I should do what he says.

But he is pulling down my pants. I should scream.

I'm paralyzed, hung between two shoulds.

Don't say anything, he says.

I should fight, I think.

I move my hips back, away from him, but his hand follows me, long finger pushes sharp into me. I scoot back until my head is hard against the wall, neck kinked.

I should fight. I put my mouth on his shoulder and bite down through his shirt. I understand all at once that he might mistake this for passion. I bite harder. I am working myself up to hurt him, I want to be ferocious, but my body hesitates. If I draw blood, if I bite right through, he will know I mean to hurt him.

I'm waiting for the certain signal that will tell me this is a fight.

He bumps his shoulder against my teeth, knocks my head against the wall.

It could have been accidental.

He drives his hand harder into me. I look down and see tendons on his wrist stand up.

His hand is violent but his face is soft, eyes rolling upward as if in prayer.

I didn't know people did this. Is this what happens between married people? All of his fingers are in me and I make a sound, an *ooph*.

The elevator comes rumbling, I can hear voices and then the ding. We both scramble. All I can think is they'll see me with my panties down, obscene. The elevator doors open and there are noisy teenage voices and thudding like when my brothers wrestle in the living room. The doors close again and it's quiet.

It's hard to do up my pants, my hands are jumping. I grab my coat and bag and fairly run for the stairs.

I'm late, I say.

He has to wait for the elevator. I get down the stairs as fast as I can, bones jittering. Out through the student union, out the doors, out.

His fingers have left a pang between my legs. I walk home feeling impeded, as though I should be the one on crutches. A long walk through the law school parking lot, cutting across the corner of Kiwanis Park, up the long hill of Apple Avenue.

I will have to tell this story again. Like Yael, I will make it into a song. In three years, I will sing this story to a courtroom.

~

Mom sinks. Job gone, she finds her place in bed. Every other week she dresses up to go to the doctor. She wants to look gorgeous, it's the only time she leaves the house anymore.

I sit cross-legged on the bed while she ransacks her closet.

This? she says, holding out a beige blouse.

No, I say. More color.

She pulls her scarf with the Mondrian colors from a drawer.

Better, I say.

Dad brought her this scarf from MoMA in New York. Mom's hands shake as she applies lipstick, leaning close to the mirror. She kisses her lips together and stands up straight, turns her shoulders flirtatiously.

I can't tell Mom about Dave H. She's too fragile to dress herself without my approval. This will shatter her. I want to believe it wasn't my fault but she will blame herself for my sin. She will ask what I was wearing and her face will go inward if I tell her about the sandals. She won't want to look at me.

One night she leaves the house, door slammed behind her, face too stunned for tears. Her car slides down the road into the night and I ask Dad where she's gone.

He rubs a finger and thumb over his eyes and says, She's trying to decide whether to kill herself.

This is surely my fault. Dad and I wait, dining room light on, we sit at the table and watch out over the valley from our giant black windows. It is morning when she comes back, her face stiff and martyred, but alive. I am twelve. I am fourteen and sixteen. I don't know how old I am.

Dad brings me to an art opening at BYU in Mom's stead. I wear a Sunday dress and put my hair up, reach out a thin arm to shake hands. I hold my cup of sparkle punch and circulate. I look at the art on the walls and push my eyebrows together and squint close at the canvas. I hold myself carefully, conscious of myself as Dad's stand-in wife.

I do Mom's laundry. The sacred garments she wears as underwear. Dad makes her dinner, serves it to her, clears her plate. All of us, all the siblings keep the house running. We are a team of wives.

Dad joins me in front of a picture and points out a technique one artist uses, explains how he's been doing the same thing over and over for years, exploring deep into that single red line that moves through all his work.

I get bored too easy for that, laughs Dad.

My sense of rightness in the church is beginning to fray. I do not belong among these righteous people. I imagine the secrets behind doors and curtained windows of our neighborhood, secrets as monstrous as mine. Almost as monstrous.

As I walk, the carillon bells chase me down the sidewalk. Every hour, they play the refrain from a hymn.

All is well, chimes the carillon.

All is well.

When I was little, we had a giant basket, big enough for me to climb into. I hauled it out to the front porch and rang the doorbell, then jumped inside, pulling the blanket up to my chin. My sister opened the door.

Oh my goodness! she said. A child!!

The happy surprise in her voice was deeply satisfying to me, it felt like falling in love would one day. I was a poor unwanted orphan left on a porch and the door opened to a flood of love and warm attention. Just like Moses in his basket of rushes, Leda in the role of the Pharaoh's daughter.

For a minute, cradled in my basket, a too-big baby, I was no longer one of the crowd. For the length of Leda's gratifying gasp, hand delicately at her breast, I was Chosen, like Moses. Like Dad chose Mom.

Fifth wiving.

Wife: girl, twelve or maybe thirteen. I'm sitting on the grass at BYU, on the slope beside the long stairway leading up from lower campus. Runners train here, puffing up and down, up and down.

Husband: I will not remember his name. My skin prickles where his arm is near mine. He is passing through town. He tells me I have pretty hair. I am awed by how grown-up he is. He touches my knuckles with one finger. A runner's shoes tap up the stairs.

The man leans in to whisper, tucks my hair behind my ear.

Would you like to come to my hotel room? he says.

Electricity crackles through me. A hotel room!

I look much older than twelve or maybe thirteen. We lie down on the hotel bed and kiss, his body touching the whole length of mine. I know I'm ruined and it doesn't matter. We keep our clothes on, mostly. He is gentle with me, his hands hovering under my shirt, above my skin. Later he writes me a letter; it goes unnoticed at home. *I asked Heaven to send Me an Angle*, he writes. *Your an Angle From Heaven like the song.* I never write him back. I'm embarrassed by his childish spelling, his sticky simplistic idealization. I'm many things, but I am not, will never be, an angel. He's a grown-up, he should be smarter than this. I'm embarrassed to have rubbed against him, to have kissed him until my lips were raw.

There will be more boys, more men, more than I can count.

It's a spring day and we're having class outside. This is MIA, Mutual Improvement Association. Years later it will be called Young Women's. At church, after sacrament meeting with everyone, and Sunday School with kids our age, the girls go to MIA and the boys to priesthood meeting. We've brought folding metal chairs to the grass so we won't ruin our Sunday clothes. This is the lesson where we're told that touching below the neck or above the knees is a sin. We are to keep ourselves pure for our future husbands; it's better to die than to lose our virtue. I am compared to a stick of gum that has been chewed and can't be unchewed. I see myself stuck to the bottom of a desk, hardened there, kids picking at me under the desk through the years. Rotten bargain for my husband-to-be. We are sitting on metal chairs in a circle, and it's a soft spring day, and I'm wearing a blue dress with little white flowers on it, and it slides over my pantyhose. I cannot look at the faces of the other girls. I am looking down at my lap, but I can see hair that has come loose and is held lightly in the breeze, sunlight making a halo of its frizzes. My memory won't tell me if this is my hair or hair belonging to the girl next to me. My memory won't give up who it is, but I can see the curve of her cheek, edged in light. We're warned about those sad girls who lose their virtue and every act that could have been loving is now rendered cheap and ugly, a trailer-trash picture conjured of a couple messing around in each others' undershirts, mouths full of the ashes of their ruined lives. I am holding the MIA manual, its slippery cover open in my lap, and there are the words, *neck* and *knees*, *below* and *above*, tight black words on a too-bright page.

Too late, I think.

Marriage rituals are tribal, strange to the uninitiated. Here in Utah you go into the temple, where only righteous adults are permitted to enter. When you emerge you are married.

Before I am born, before my brothers and my sister exist, Mom and Dad walk out the St. George Temple door into red-dirt desert. Both in their traveling suits, hers glowing white against the red rocks. Dad with a wide monkey grin. They climb into their decorated car. Driver's side labeled *Him*, passenger *Her*. The rear door reads, *Vacancy*.

Streamers streaming, they speed off to copulate. We are a half step away from the bloody sheet as evidence of virginity.

PART 2: TEEN BRIDE

I, the Lord God, delight in the chastity of women.

Jacob 2:28, *Book of Mormon*

1983

I LEAN CLOSE TO THE mirror, paint a single black line along my top eyelid and long beyond the corner of my eye, winged up at the end like ballet stage makeup. I've become expert after years of recitals, Nutcrackers, Coppelias. Another line below my bottom lashes. The line jogs and I have to start over, steady the heel of my hand against my chin. I am wearing a brother's old Boy Scout shirt and a plaid Catholic schoolgirl miniskirt. I swiped the skirt from the costume shop at Provo High. My friend Anika and I work there, a cramped space above the stage. I shook dust out of the skirt, held it up to my hips.

Keep? I asked.

Definitely, she said.

I touch my face carefully. My lips are cracked and peeled beyond their natural border. I was cursed with Jobian boils like Mom had once, her soft skin now cratered with scars. Now I'm part of clinical trials for a new acne drug. I've just finished a course and my skin is beginning to heal.

I'm fifteen and still in the habit of seeing myself as hideous.

Today after third period, a junior blocks my way in Main Hall. He is soft around the middle and I have a small crush on him. He carries a half-smile on his face like he appreciates the irony of our entire high school world.

Are you ticklish? he asks.

Don't even try it, I say.

Come on now.

Don't. Don't.

He has his hands on me and he's tickling, hard. I can't get away. He's just playing. Other kids are watching. He can't know the trapped-animal feeling that rises in me.

I said NO.

My knee flashes upward, faster than consciousness. I get him right in the balls.

He's on the floor, dropped like a sack of bricks. His friends back away, a space opens around us. I'd heard about kicking a boy in the balls, but I'd never seen what it could do. His face is as red as an infant struggling for enough breath to cry.

I'm sorry I'm sorry, I say.

I reach down to help him up but he shoots me a bright, hateful look.

I back away. I'm shaking with leftover anger, fear. The boy is slowly getting to his feet.

I didn't mean it, I say.

But I did mean it. I meant it and I am monstrous. Now he's broken and it's my fault.

When he sees me in the halls after, he'll put his hands up like a boxer and laugh, but his cheeks will flush. We will be too embarrassed to speak to each other anymore.

Sixth, seventh wiving.

Eighth wiving, ninth.

I've lost track.

I've crashed a Halloween dance at BYU. I'm using a fake French accent; I think this will make me interesting.

At the dance is a college guy in a bowler hat, T-shirt, and suit jacket. Patrick. He asks me to dance.

He reminds me of the guy from school, the one I knee in the balls. But Patrick's ironic amusement is more convincing, he's had time to shape it.

I give him my number. He calls later in the week. I'm in my sister's old room, now remade as a library.

On the phone I come clean.

I'm not French, I say.

His laugh is wide open, he loves the joke. I wind myself in the looped phone cord as we talk. We talk for an hour, two.

My first date with Patrick is a double feature at BYU's international cinema. I tell my parents I'm meeting my friend Mary. I will not be allowed to date until I'm sixteen, and a twenty-two-year-old man is out of the question anyway.

I get to the cinema and he doesn't show. The movie starts, and still no Patrick. I call him from the phone down the hall. He forgot about our date but says he'll be over soon, we can watch the second movie. He appears with his *Norton Anthology of Literature* in hand, an absurdly thick book, dog-eared. We walk along the winding paths through the botanical gardens as it starts to get dark. I stand close to him under a street light, he reads me poetry, resting the book awkwardly against his belly.

There are emergency phones in pools of light at intervals along the pathways.

At Provo High, we call these the Rape Paths.

The second feature is about to start, Patrick and I hurry back. We walk into the theater holding hands, fresh from the outside, and I am fizzy with romance. Something at the edge of my vision snags my attention:

Dad.

He is standing at the back of the theater, arms folded. My heart slams my ribs.

Mary, it seems, called me at home, all innocent.

Dad grips my elbow hard, like I'm a naughty toddler. He pulls me out of the theater, leaving Patrick alone to watch *Forbidden Games*.

I sluff class at Provo High to meet Patrick in the student union, the same building where I met Dave H. He's waiting for me on the third floor, under the pictures of BYU beauty queens. He sits on a bench, elbows on his knees.

Above his head is a picture of a woman I know from the neighborhood, when she was a student. She is tinted in pinks and blues, looks up and to the right of the frame, into the future. Now she has a mess of kids and sells real estate.

I sit next to him. We talk, we flirt, our words run out and we are quiet and then he stands. He holds a hand out to me and pulls me close. He tips his head to the right. A small kiss, held for two seconds, and then he puts his arms around me. He laughs quietly in my ear.

I can't believe I just kissed a fifteen-year-old, he says.

When he kisses me again I'm hungry, I put my fingers on his shirt and take his tongue into my mouth.

This is our secret.

He lives in the finished basement of his parents' house. We sit on the low couch and he hands me a cup of hot chocolate.

Have you ever had rum? he asks.

I shake my head. I've never had any alcohol.

He produces a bottle, pours it into my hot chocolate. I drink, he refills our mugs, refills again. He shows me his bedroom, the computer at the desk.

This, he says, is called a *mouse*.

We make squeaking sounds.

A mouse! I say.

I start to laugh, fumble my way out to the couch, laughing, until rum and hot chocolate rumble up my throat, I laugh it all onto his rug, I'm on my knees, a hand over my mouth.

Oh, I say. I'm sorry, I say.

It's okay, he says. His voice smiles, indulgent. He brings a washcloth to clean the carpet. The stain will never come out. Every time I go to his house, I will see the shape of my vomit.

Tonight, drunk, I sit on the floor and lean my head against his legs. He's talking and I am warm under the blanket he brought from his room.

I'm agnostic, he says.

I'd read the word, but never heard anyone use it. It's really possible, I think, to just not believe.

Maybe I don't believe either. There's no home for me in the Church, I've known this for a while. No place for me in Heavenly Father's Celestial Kingdom.

I sluff school almost every day, meet Patrick on campus. I sit in on his poetry class, in back. The professor is from Wales, thinning red hair and blue eyes that are wide as though he sees God. He recites *The Waste Land*, thundering:

Burning burning burning burning

O Lord, thou pluckest me out

O Lord, thou pluckest

Burning

I'm burning for Patrick when we meet beneath the homecoming queens, burning when he smuggles me into his car, burning when we go to the park. We sit on the grass and he leans against a tree.

When you're eighteen, he says, We'll make love for the first time here, between these two trees.

In his basement room, he pins a quote from *A Midsummer Night's Dream* to his bulletin board:

O spite, too old to be engag'd to young!

We'll never get married, he says. Marriage is for people who need a piece of paper to prove their love. We'll live together, he says, but never marry.

Mom is embroidering a green satin temple apron. She's on her way down from peak Heavy, beginning to stir herself. She's on the bed but not under the covers, a good sign.

The apron symbolizes the fig leaves Adam and Eve used to cover their nakedness. At a certain point in the temple ceremony, attendees tie these aprons over their white temple clothes. The aprons are meant to be simple. They are all made to the same template, no variation allowed.

But you can embroider it, says Mom. With green thread only.

Mom tells me this as she embroiders. I'm too young to go to the temple. She isn't supposed to reveal its secrets, but she tells me bits and pieces.

I think you would appreciate the symbolism, she says. It is strange and beautiful.

Mom is pushing the boundaries of what is allowed. Her green-on-green embroidery admits a narrow space for her eccentricity, the outlines of the leaves swooped and shaped into baroque scallops. This apron is a gift for my brother's fiancée—she'll wear it when she marries my brother.

At its core, Mormonism is a mystical religion. I picture the temple ceremony, white-costumed believers sweeping their arms in choreographed signs, aprons unfolded in unison to hide their figurative nakedness.

Mom's needle moves in and out, she pulls shining green thread taut, hands making semaphores. The apron on her lap, she on the king-size bed under Dad's angel painting. The angel looks down on Mom, paused in flight. He is somehow feral, scaled up from human size just enough to be disturbing.

I think of myself as an apostate. This is my secret.

Dave H appears at my high school. It's been years, but I recognize him. At first only his silhouette in the glass door at the back of A Wing. He is tall, hair still feathered to his collar. I know it's him before I see his face. A grown-up man walking down the hall with a girl I know, Angel.

My body moves before my brain catches up. I hop out of sight, then speed down Main Hall. I want space. I don't look behind me. I just keep moving until I'm at the far end of the hall and then I bust out through the doors to the parking lot.

He didn't see me he didn't see me, I think.

My whole body is shaking.

It's the next day when I see Angel again. She's at her locker and I am close beside her in the almost-shelter of her locker door. I tell her to stay away from Dave H. When she asks why, I tell her the story. She's the first person I've told. I was so proud I'd been able to hold this inside me for years, but I'd kept from myself that he was still out there. He is a loaded gun. If I deserved it, Angel doesn't.

In class the next day, I'm paged over the intercom. *Amie Myer to the Principal's office.* I can feel my pulse in my teeth. The Principal's office never holds good news. The secretary hands me the phone over her high counter. It's Dad on the phone. He got a call from BYU police. Angel must have called them.

Amie, he says. Is it true?

I can't see anything in front of me. I am taking a step into the void.

Yes, I say.

You're sure, he says. It really happened?

He doesn't believe me, I think. I doubt myself.

It really happened, I say.

I'm sorry, I say.

Oh Amie, he says. I picture him, holding the phone with one hand, the other moving up and over his bald head.

> *Blessed above women shall Jael the wife of Heber the Kenite be, blessed shall she be above women in the tent.*

In court, I raise one hand, finger pointed.

I point at Dave H in his orange jumpsuit.

In court, I say *He unbuttoned my pants.*

His blond hair is a nimbus of sunlight.

In court, he looks at me and I look at him.

I lift a hand and point at him.

In court, I say *It took him ten seconds to open my pants.*

I do not know how long it took.

In court, I say *He put his fingers inside me.*

I remember how it felt, his fingers stabbed.

In court, I say *It was him.*

Can you show us who it was? says the attorney.

In court, I lift a hand.

I stab my finger at him.

She put her hand to the nail, and her right hand to the workmen's hammer; and with the hammer she smote Sisera, she smote off his head, when she had pierced and stricken through his temples.

At her feet he bowed, he fell, he lay down: at her feet he bowed, he fell: where he bowed, there he fell down dead.

He is not convicted. It would have been a miracle if he had been. Nearly three years after the fact, no evidence. But but, I think. A policewoman went undercover and he tried the same thing with her. That had to count for something.

It didn't. It counted for nothing.

In Utah, twelve is old enough to consent to almost anything. Not intercourse. Not penis-in-vagina, no, but to anything else a twelve-year-old can say, Yes, I want to do that.

He never denied it happened. He just said I wanted it.

Did I? Have I been telling myself a false story all these years?

He knows where I live. He'll be mad at me. I put this whole machine in motion, police and lawyers and a courtroom full of people, I wasted all their time, exhausted all their spirits.

I want to forget he ever existed.

Outside the courtroom, Dad is shrunk, his eyebrows disarranged. This is my fault, too.

He and I do not talk about it. My mother never asks about any of it, not about the assault, not about court. I'm not entirely sure Dad told her, and I certainly won't. She is too precarious.

We spend our days weaving a protective shell around Mom in her bedroom, we keep her shielded from all the noise of living.

It's my sixteenth birthday: I'm able to date for real. All boys at my birthday party except my best friend, Anika. Halfway through the video of *Zelig* she climbs to the roof to make out with a boy. On the kitchen counter is a calendar and a pen; boys are to claim a day on the calendar for a date with me. It's not serious, it's a terrific joke, it's deadly serious. I might in fact have signed up half a dozen boys, but I only remember one. Joe from Salt Lake City will take me to Applebee's on his motorcycle, my first official, parent-sanctioned date. He's twenty years old but at least he's going through proper channels. He will wear a suit and I a white dress, and the waitress will think we are a married couple on an anniversary date. We marry young around here. After dinner a ride up Provo Canyon into green night, and I'll burn my bare calf on his exhaust. But I am not a wuss, I'm game, I won't ruin the evening. He'll give me his suit jacket against the cold and trees will shush by, and in my memory we will be the only people on the road.

At my birthday party, next to the calendar, is a bouquet of red roses from Patrick, who is in Santa Cruz for the summer. *The botanical beauties, thirteen in number, represent the asymmetry I prize in you, as well as the conventions we cheerfully mock with our love,* he wrote in the card. It's true, it's all true, I love Patrick, and it's a great and forbidden love, and I ride a nighttime motorcycle with Salt Lake Joe, and I'm sixteen and surrounded by boys, and we all knew this is who I always was.

Wife: sixteen-year-old me.

A friend at school tells me there's a party and she can't go but I should. She writes the address on a scrap of notebook paper.

It's an apartment near BYU, one of the long low apartment complexes. My sister lived in one across the street when she first got married.

Husband: the guy who opens the door is hard, handsome in a way that does not belong to Utah Valley. His T-shirt pulls tight over muscles. I'm embarrassed at my teenager body, thrift store punk clothes. I give my friend's name as my pass. His face opens to an easy smile, he steps back to show me into the apartment.

Nobody else is here.

You're early, he says. My roommate went to get stuff for the party.

Come on in, he says. I'm watching a movie.

I follow him down the hall to his room. He sits on the bed and pats the space next to him. *Scarface* is on TV. He tells me he's seventeen, but he's very tall, very broad.

Later I will learn he is lying about his age, and his name. He's in his twenties.

Want some gum? he says.

He smiles and goosebumps trill my skin. That sickish plumbline drop from throat to belly. I take the gum and I think I smile but my face is numb. I imagine kissing him. I imagine looking at him over pizza at the party, his private smile just for me. I imagine him laughing at something I say, leaning in to whisper *You're so cute* in my ear.

And then he's on me. His kiss smashes my lips against my teeth. I'm pulling back, it's too hard too quick, but he pushes me down on the bed.

I think if he touches my breasts it will be okay. It's too fast but okay, I can be okay. He is not interested in the top half of my body. He flips up my skirt and yanks down my underwear and I'm naked from the waist down, which feels more naked, ugly. We've skipped ahead somewhere. We were flirting. I let him kiss me.

I don't know what I missed.

Don't say anything, he says.

It's the same thing Dave H said. They have the same script.

My tongue is hard on my palate, I'm making a *nnnnnn* sound, I mean it to be *No*, but it comes out deflated. *Nnnnn-uh.*

I don't know what I could say. There's nobody here but him.

I push his shoulders away from me. I can't convince my voice to make a full *No* but I am pushing him away. My teeth are closed tightly together, I'm breathing heavily through my nose. My jaw will hurt later. It's work. I'm wrestling this man on top of me and it is terrifyingly impersonal. He uses his knees to push my legs apart like it's manual labor, he's just doing his job. No sound but my breath, his, bed springs, bodies thudding mattress.

He has his penis in his hand, pushes it bluntly into me. I'm trying to lift myself onto my elbows but his weight pushes me into the bed. I try to crabwalk my bottom but he is stuck hard to me. I just want a minute, I just want to catch up.

I wonder if I will bleed on his sheets.

I didn't tell him I was a virgin, I think.

I don't know what the protocol is. I don't know if it's polite to tell your rapist it's your first time. I'm embarrassed. I don't want him to see my blood. I don't want him to think I'm on my period. I don't want him to be disgusted by me.

We struggle together. He holds my hair in one hand, pulled back so I can't bring my chin down. It's hard to swallow. I don't know if he knows he's hurting me.

He must not know, I think.

If he knew, he'd stop, I think.

I am not going to cry, I think.

I'm not a wuss, I think. I'm not a crybaby.

I can handle this, I think.

He's all the way inside me and then it feels like his penis kinks, hard against my inside wall. This hurts more than anything that came before and my breath chokes in my throat and he makes a surprised bark in my ear.

Does it hurt him, too?

I want to say *I'm sorry* but I can't get any breath behind the words.

The way he's holding my hair, my face is tipped up and back toward the bedroom door. It's open. I am terribly sure his roommate will appear in the doorway with groceries, party supplies. Any second.

Please please don't let a stranger see me like this.

Afterward he drives me home. I don't ask if there was ever meant to be a party. It's not until later that I realize I shouldn't have told him where I live. Something seeps between my legs.

I will leave a bloodstain on the passenger seat, I think.

Later I will wonder if I bled at all, it seems absurd that I would after all my wickedness, *virgin* hardly seemed the right word for me anyway. I didn't check the sheets. My underwear was missing. I was getting dressed without looking at him, without looking at anything. I was getting dressed and laughing shakily like *Oh haha, aren't we a crazy couple of kids?*

Wetness between the thighs will become familiar, but for now I think it's blood.

I picture him on his knees, car door open, scrubbing and scrubbing. The mark will pale but its outlines will stay. My humiliating revenge.

In the car he jokes about having just raped me. He covers my knee with his hand, laughing.

I'm not such a bad guy, he says. Rapists don't give rides home. Ha ha!

I am arguing with myself.

This was your fault, I think. You went to his apartment. You had twenty boys at your birthday party. You wanted him to kiss you, even though you love Patrick. You didn't scream. You didn't bite and scratch and fight. *It is better to die in defending one's virtue*, wrote our prophet, President Kimball, *than to live having lost it without a struggle.*

It couldn't be rape.

I was ready to die, I think.

(But I was afraid to hurt him.)

It was rape, I think. It was.

Better dead than unclean is just Mormon crap, I think.

I'm an apostate anyway.

Nobody can know, I think. Mom will break.

I saw how reduced Dad was in court, his expression helpless, the giant-like strength of my childhood Dad flaking away in layers.

Mom will break all the way down, I think.

I'm at the pay phone just outside school. I lift the heavy phone book in its metal cradle. My finger on the entry: Rape Crisis.

I'll just ask, I think. I won't give my name, I think. All I want, I think, is to find out how this works.

It isn't just my parents who need protection. The man, too. His hand on my knee. He wanted my forgiveness. We are supposed to forgive. If I go to the police he'll think I mean to hurt him.

Pointing at Dave H in court was an act of violence. I pointed at him and he saw me point, he saw my face and he knows my name.

One ring, two. I let the phone book swing down into place.

Rape Crisis, says a voice.

I think I've been raped, I say into the phone.

Okay, says the woman. Have you been to the hospital?

No, I say. Can we do this without telling my parents?

Not if you want to report it to the police.

No police, I say.

I have no control over my voice, it wobbles high.

The rape crisis woman meets me at the hospital. I've told her she can recognize me from my long black coat with the black-and-white checked lining.

I'm put in a room, exam table, my feet up in the stirrups. I didn't know exam tables came with these. They keep them tucked away, hidden like the nail file in a Swiss army knife.

I've never had a pelvic exam before. Rapecrisis Woman sits on a chair to my right. I think of this as her name, better as a name than the words *rape* and *crisis*.

My legs wide open to the door, I'm naked from the waist down like the nightmare where you've forgotten your pants. My knees drift toward each other but with my feet like this I can't close them. A person in blue scrubs opens the door and turns quick to the left, then right. He does not look at me. Ducking like he can hide his face behind his clipboard. I crunch the blue paper down between my legs and try to sit up. He tells Rapecrisis Woman that they can't do the exam without parental permission.

I can't tell my parents, I say, my voice too loud.

The man in scrubs looks at me like he's just noticed I'm there. He shakes his head. There's nothing he can do.

Rapecrisis Woman leaves me some privacy to get dressed. I have a hectic time getting back into my clothes. I don't know what to do next. Rapecrisis Woman came all this way to help me, I can't let it stop here.

Back out in the waiting room, Rapecrisis Woman looks at me, eyebrows raised.

I'm sorry, she says. She lifts her hands, drops them at her sides.

I know another doctor, I say. My family doctor.

I've been seeing him since I was a kid. At his office, Dr. Swell gravely agrees to see me without a signature from Dad. I won't know until many years later that this is a risk for him. He's supposed to report rape. He's not supposed to treat me without parental permission. But he steps quietly out of the room while I get undressed for the second time today.

Another exam table, stirrups. My family doctor down there between my knees. He has to tell me to keep my knees apart, to scoot down on the table so I'm splayed wide open. My mind flashes for a second to the bed at the not-party. My knees are shaking but the doctor's voice is steady. Rapecrisis Woman asks if I want to hold her hand.

Can I?

The speculum slides into me, locks open. I breathe in sharp, did not know there would be things prying me open like this.

And then the lights go out.

Power outage, says Dr. Swell. He pauses for just a minute. I laugh into the darkness. On my back, knees open, and now the power goes out. Too much.

Listen, he says. If it's all right with you, I'm going to keep going. Don't want to make this last any longer than it has to. Just give me half a minute.

I see a flashlight wobble over the walls. Tighten my grip on Rapecrisis Woman's hand.

Okay, he says. You have tearing inside.

It's real, I think. I didn't make this up. There's a man in a white coat, an authority, and he is pronouncing it real. Here is evidence. A great rush of relief moves through me.

This woman I've never met before and the doctor who treated my childhood earaches are caring for me like parents.

The rest is bearable. The giant Q-tip that fingers my cervix and kicks up an odd nausea. The speculum unlatching and sliding out. The lights flood on just before he inserts the needle to take my blood. We all laugh softly as he clicks off the flashlight.

I've gotten dressed and I'm standing at the high desk for my bill. I can't pay now, but I ask them to send me the bill, put my name on the envelope, please, not my dad's. I'm working out numbers in my head, I'll pay it off a little at a time.

And then I black out. Not a picturesque crumple to the ground. I topple like a board. Know nothing until I'm looking at Rapecrisis Woman from the floor. The look on her face is cartoonish surprise. I start to laugh. I'm lying on the floor and cracking up at all of it, monstrously absurd. When I get to my feet we're all laughing, relief in Rapecrisis Woman's face, the receptionist, the doctor. I hold onto the high desk like I'm trying to stay upright on a pitching ship, the weirdest most hilarious terrible day of my life so far.

The doctor never sends a bill, never tells my parents. Twenty-five years later I'll get a copy of my medical records and see his notes. RAPE will be written in block letters across the top. I'll crack wide open then, grieve all of it for the first time.

This will seem like piling on. It strains credulity, I don't seem credible, not even to myself. This can't be how the world works, the story has no space for it.

And, also, there is something pornographic in these stories. That slick, creeping feeling, this is woman at her most elemental, stripped and opened to a man.

I am going along with my high school life, *until*.

I want him to kiss me.

He gives me gum.

He kisses me.

He lays me back on his bed.

Scarface is on TV.

I didn't tell him I'm a virgin, I think.

I always tell the truth, says Al Pacino. *Even when I lie.*

Shhhh, he says.

Blessed shall she be above women in the tent.

His face is too close to bear.

Behind him, Al Pacino explodes with a gun, an orgy of blood.

He asked water, and she gave him milk.

To be a good girl, I should fight.

. . . with the hammer she smote Sisera, she smote off his head.

To be a good wife, I should help him.

Instead, I am an animal who is attacked and shows its belly.

I am an animal who freezes.

I freeze.

It sounds so simple. Fight back. Die rather than be raped. But this is a person I'm naked with. My brain says naked = intimate. I think it's easy to die. I've talked with death since I was seven. It's hard to hurt someone. It's hard to risk dislike. Kill me, but don't dislike me. Rape me, don't dislike me. Love me. Love me. Love me. I don't care how you show it.

I've cut off all my hair, buzzed it down to a flattop. Mom locks herself in her bathroom to cry. She's in there over an hour. When she opens the door, she tells me my flattop is slutty.

No, you don't understand, I say. The Farrah flip is slutty. Not this.

We both know we have to navigate the complicated, ever-changing codes of womanhood. We both fail, in our separate ways.

Why do you wear such baggy clothes? says Mom. Don't hide that tight little body of yours.

Patrick has fallen off his scooter and broken his wrist, has to have surgery. I go to see him in the hospital, walk into his room with a rose. He is in bed in his hospital gown and he takes the rose and puts it between his teeth. He lifts one eyebrow at me, then the other, laughs the rose out of his mouth. I put the rose in a cup of water, sit on the bed. He kisses me and slides his hands under my shirt. He touches my breast with just the fingers of his broken hand, the rest of it mummied in bandages that rough my nipple.

When you're eighteen, he starts to say, like we often say.

We don't have to wait, I say.

His bandaged hand stops.

It's okay, I say. I'm not a virgin anymore.

He pulls his hand away and sits back against his pillow while I tell him the story. I don't tell him the part where I wanted the man to kiss me. He doesn't ask any questions. He shakes his head and rubs his eyes and then he rings for the nurse.

I want to tell him everything but now is not the time.

I wait while Patrick heals. Tonight we are in line to see *Nosferatu*. It's Halloween, our one-year anniversary. His hand is out of its cast, an ugly scar running around his thumb.

I want him to know I was really raped, the doctor said so. I tell him about the doctor because if Patrick can understand, it means I didn't ask for it. I want him to absolve me. But he lets go of my hand and shakes his head, he shakes it in a very big *No No No*, and it's clear. This is not something I should talk about.

If it happens to a girl once, says a friend at school, okay, she was raped. But more than that, and it's her fault.

I feel violently out of sync with the sunlight world.

Tearing inside is not enough. I want bruises. I want broken bones. I want visible evidence. My unmarked body, the tight body Mom wants me to show off, accuses me.

It's night and I'm in my bedroom with a hard-backed hymnal. I'm working up my nerve. I bring the hymnal to eye-level, then slam it into my face. I slam the hymnal over and over until I see stars. But I pull my punches just enough, hesitate before the blow. Like I hesitated my teeth on Dave H's shoulder. I inspect myself in the mirror. One eye, one cheek is red, but I know it's not enough. Any bruise will be slight. I shake my head at myself. Always overdramatizing things.

Coward, I think.

I have a history test in the morning, and I haven't studied. I don't think I even have the book. I've been spinning for a while now. I sign Mom's name better than she does. *Please excuse my daughter, who is ill.* Sluff more classes than I attend.

Maybe it's history. Maybe biology. Doesn't matter. Revulsion, terror move through my body. I can't face it. I can't walk into class tomorrow and stare at the test and fail.

I used to be the heroine of my own story. The kidnapped girl who knocks her captors unconscious and makes her escape, bloody and barely clothed. Picture on the front page: *Girl Foils Kidnappers.*

Kidnappers would be clear. Kidnappers would hold a gun to my head, no mistake, the borders sharply drawn. Not this dripping, womanish shame.

I kneel on the floor of my bedroom, fold forward over my legs. I prostrate myself.

Please, I say. I don't know who I'm begging: deity, parents, me. I want absolution but I don't know how to ask. Only *Please. Please.* Hysteria rises and I whisper-howl into the carpet, Violent Femmes on the tape player. They spit angry lyrics while I'm twisting on the ancient green shag of my bedroom floor.

I want to be angry. *You can all just kiss off into the air.* I want to stir myself into anger pure as the music but all I have is this girlish weakness, I'm only angry at myself. The tape clicks off.

Sudden, perfect quiet. It's three in the morning, the house in black sleep.

A solution creeps into my mind. I will fix everything. All the tension slides from my body, and I stretch out on the floor, eye-level with the green shag.

I listen to my breath.

In the morning, I take two bottles from my mom's medicine cabinet, tuck them into my book bag. Also my copy of Shakespeare, *Complete Works*. I put a bookmark in the *Out, out, brief candle* soliloquy.

When I'm grown, I'll be embarrassed by this. I picked something that obvious.

None of my friends have any beer or wine or Everclear in their locker, today of all days. Coca-Cola will have to do—caffeine is bad for you, right. So maybe that will help the pills along. I go to the seminary building, settle on the couch outside the classrooms. I want to make some kind of statement, something about hypocrisy and the church. I am not allowed into the temple. The best I can do is a taupe couch on beige carpet, teenagers passing with leather-bound scriptures.

Later I will make a joke about half-assing my own suicide. Close-enoughing it like a late book report. Coca-Cola, Excedrin PM, and Shakespeare.

But I've already half-stepped out of life. I feel unburdened, free as a little kid. I'll finish and none of this has anything to do with me. Not anymore.

I gag a couple of times on the pills, but I get them down, I manage. And then I lie down and wait.

In the thin pre-sleep space between thought and dream, I feel a hand on my shoulder. I turn to the hand in my almost-dream. Another hand, another. I'm pulled upright. My eyes open but I can't focus. I'm on the couch. Seminary building. In front of me are faces.

Jack. Sean. Friends.

I feel my eyes rolling away. Jack shakes me.

Wake up, he says.

No, I say. Let me sleep.

I lean sideways but they don't let me lie down.

Nope, says Sean.

They pull me to standing. Jack holds me while Sean puts my crutches under my arms. I squint down at the crutches. Tore my ligaments my first time on skis, what, last week? The week before?

Come on, says Jack. We're going for a walk.

I'm shaking my head but they laugh.

Later they will tell me they didn't know why they did this. Later I'll be told that if I'd slipped all the way into sleep, that would have been it, I'd have been done. Excedrin PM was the real thing in 1984. Caffeine, it turns out, was a good accelerant toward the big sleep.

Sean and Jack walk me out of the seminary building and into the main school building.

I lean my head against Jack's shoulder, and he pushes it back upright. Sean, on my right, is kicking my good foot forward.

Look, I say. Stop. Stop.

They don't stop. My vision has black fog around the edges, like a photo vignette. I have to concentrate very hard to make words.

I'm *trying*, I say. I don't finish this sentence. Tears leak out of my eyes.

Look, I say again. Okay. I took some pills. I want to go to sleep.

There it is. I tell on myself. Sean holds me up while Jack goes for the school counselor.

I am exhausted, desperate to sleep, but a voice keeps pulling at me—someone's talking and I want to let unconsciousness take me but I can't. The voice escalates from nails-on-a-blackboard annoyance to scraping my bones, it won't fucking stop.

I'm sitting in the counselor's office. My dad is here, talking talking.

It's your obsession with boys, says Dad.

I lean over and vomit into the wastebasket. Next thing I'm in the waiting room at the doctor's office. It's clear across town from school, but the ride in the car is gone, wiped from my tapes. There are coughing kids in the waiting room. Flu season. I'm folded over in my chair, head on my knees. I vomit again. I don't know if it makes it into the wastebasket, but this gets me into a room quick. The paper on the exam table is crackling beneath me and here's Dr. Swell.

He looks so sad.

He tells my father to take me to the emergency room. I feel like I'm laughing, but I don't know if it shows on the outside. The emergency room is all the way across town again, over by Provo High. I want to say this stopped being an emergency hours ago, but it's back in the car and then I'm ralphing in the hospital parking lot.

A woman with long braids tells me it's good I threw up so much; they won't have to pump my stomach. She's maybe twenty years old. Holds a stack of papers, asks me a long list of questions. Just when I think she's done, she turns to a new page. None of these questions seem relevant, and I don't know where my dad is.

Do *you* hear voices? I ask her.

Ha ha, she says.

And then I'm in the juvenile psych ward, fifth floor. I'm put into bed and finally I can sleep. It's dark when I wake up. The air smells like a TV dinner. A nurse is in my room, whispering to someone else. I pretend I'm having a horrifying nightmare. I know I'm being watched and I perform, squirm in bed. I know they see through it. It's humiliating. I know this, and I amp up the show, writhe in the sheets, whimper.

In the morning my friend Missy is sitting on a bed kitty-corner to mine. The last time I saw her was at an abandoned house across the street from school. Graffiti all over the walls. We were talking casually about breaking the windows and she turned and punched her bare hand through one.

According to kids at school, she was possessed by the Devil. The Elders were giving her a blessing—they commanded the demon to leave her body and she threw one of the Elders across the room. Missy can't be more than ninety-eight pounds. I don't ask if it's true.

I thought she was in Idaho.

She hugs me around the neck and then a man in baggy pants gives me the tour. I'm not sure who he is; he wears no scrubs, no lab coat, no badge that I can see. Bathrooms. Seclusion, with carpeted walls. The big room for group therapy. Boys' wing (not allowed to enter). Snack room. He tells me they have just installed windows with a special film, I can't break through them—even if I throw a brick, it'll just bounce off.

So don't get any ideas, he says. He hands me off to a nurse and I never see him again.

Missy is cross-legged on my bed when I get back.

Toilet paper's rationed, she says. The toilet backs up almost every day.

She makes a face. She looks like she should be in an ad, fresh-faced blonde, girl next door.

No shoelaces, no razors, she says. You have to use an electric razor to shave your legs.

She looks down to pick at the bedspread, and the curve of her neck knocks my heart. So beautiful. I'm really alive, then.

The hospital is Spirit Prison. Not earth with its gangs of preppies, its lockers and classrooms. Not heaven, not Outer Darkness. A waiting room for souls until Armageddon. At dinnertime Missy and I walk to the cafeteria. Teen patients are lined up in front of the window for their meds. They stand and wait.

We are souls in waiting, between worlds. This suits me fine.

Missy is on her way out. I've only been here a few days before she is packing her bag. We hug hard and I think I'll never see her again; she'll slip back into the world and my mind cannot imagine anything further ahead than snack time.

Dad sends clothes and my tape player. A Chopin tape Patrick made for me. At the end of the summer, just after he got back from Santa Cruz, we had a picnic in the mountains and he brought a boombox and champagne. I was in charge of lunch, brought Styrofoam containers of messy Hawaiian food—rice and barbequed ribs.

Patrick opened his and laughed quietly, then looked at me and laughed bigger. He lay back in the grass and let his laugh climb the canyon walls.

I thought you'd get, you know. Baguettes and cheese, he said.

I don't know where to get baguettes, I said. Anyway, this is my favorite.

We got drunk and, with Chopin playing, he lifted my shirt and my bare breasts were against his chest. I straddled his lap, my front to his, and he put his fingers inside me and I jumped and sucked air through my teeth and he held his hand still, he kissed me until I began to move, minutely. It was ter-rible, and my body wanted it. Afterward I was sore and shamed.

Tonight after lights out, I put the tape player under my pillow, volume as low as possible. Then the crescendo. Piano smashes into the dark and—

Aaarrgh! says a roommate.

Turn it down! says another.

No, you don't understand, I say. It's classical. If I turn it down I can't hear the pianissimo parts.

Fuck off, says a roommate.

I click the tape off. I lie on my back, eyes open, alone in the dark.

Dad comes to see me in the hospital. He sits on my bed and pulls out a sheet of paper and a charcoal pencil.

Do you know how to draw a face? he asks.

I shrug. Kind of.

So you draw an oval first, right? he says. He is drawing as he speaks.

And then you can rough in the features, he says. He draws a rounded cross that meets in the middle of the oval.

The eyes, he says, are halfway down the face.

No way, I say.

It's true. We're all forehead. Me especially, he says laughing, rubbing his hand over his bald head. He leaves a streak of charcoal on his skull.

He shows me how to draw eyes, nose, mouth. I will remember this lesson, use it when drawing, for the rest of my life.

After a couple weeks, I get a few hours' leave. Dad takes me to the gallery at BYU. A show is up. Dad has several pieces in it, his Emperor Hirohito painting, which fills an entire wall and rocks my eyes right open. Mostly his abstract expressionist stuff. And one piece I don't recognize. The canvas is broad and shallow, nine feet wide. It's mostly white, all negative space. A rope dangles from the top of the frame, an actual rope. The painting itself shows a figure collapsed in the far corner, she is distant in an empty room.

Is that—? I say. I don't want to assume it's me.

It's about the whole experience, says Dad. He's not looking at me.

Your mom hates it, he says. She doesn't want it in the house.

It looks like me, it looks the way I want Dad to see me, a whole person with her own inner world, isolated and damaged but still alive. It's wrong but I love this piece so much.

Like Mom in her bed. Or Dad's crucifixion painting. Jesus safely nailed to the cross, where we're happy to keep him; a god who is free and burning with power is terrifying. He's in white space too, but he fills it, hands big as houses. Jesus right up in your face. In mine, you have to travel miles to reach me across all that white. But we're both pinned in place. All of us. Mom under the pushing hand of the bedroom angel and me in a far corner and Jesus hammered to his cross.

My cousin, the cousin whose lap I climbed into when I was seven, learns I'm in the hospital. He gets permission to see me. He's in his twenties now, married. We meet in Seclusion, the room with carpeted walls. One of the boys here had to stay the night in Seclusion, and we all heard him, tossing himself over and over into the walls.

They've set up folding chairs in here for us. We sit facing each other. He's tall and he's got a ski tan. Wears his concerned look. He asks how I'm doing. I teenage-shrug at him. He tells me he's sorry I'm here. I don't know what he means by coming here. I mean, he does concerned really well. He often talks to me in that gentle, *I'm telling you this for your own good* voice, but it isn't like he's all that old. He folds his arms over his chest and stretches his legs out long in front of him. My heart gets fat in my chest.

I love him, I think.

Being in the psych ward confers a certain invulnerability. I'm not out there in the world. I can handle here. Mentally ill kids are much more direct than kids on the outside. The power balance has shifted toward me. And I'm zipped open with group therapy and family therapy and individual therapy. I'm saying it almost before I can think about it.

I don't know if it's only a dream or what, I say. I don't know if it actually happened.

He pulls his legs in.

Sits up in his chair.

I feel an electric wave move through my body.

I love him but I can't live in not-knowing anymore. A couple of weeks ago I tried to kill myself, but this is scarier.

Easier to die than to hurt someone.

Easier to die than be disliked.

We are staring at each other. He's not going to be the one to say it. Has to be me.

Did it happen? I say. When I was little. Did you—?

Yes, he says. Nodding fast. He starts to cry.

I'm sorry, he says. I'm sorry.

Thank you, he says.

I don't know if either of us says the word *molested*. I don't know if we talk about the mechanics of what happened. Maybe I ask if his wife knows, but I can't swear to it. We are both red-faced and drowningly embarrassed. I am picturing him in his boxer shorts, his hand on mine. He thanks me for asking him, thanks me for bringing it up. He talks about his sin. He begs me to forgive him.

Of course, I say quickly.

He didn't deny any of it. I am validated.

He says *It happened*. He says *Forgive me*, and already he's disappearing from the story. It isn't about him anymore. It's done and forgiven and this is supposed to wipe it all out. I will keep it secret because he owned up, and so in the same moment it's real, it is also entirely mine. A magic trick. It is very heavy, this thing. It pulls on me, and I am not feeling very strong. I keep thinking now I should be over it. Forgiveness asked and given, now I can put it away.

For thirty years I will think this.

Then she came to the pillar of the bed, which was at Holofernes' head . . .

And approached to his bed, and took hold of the hair of his head, and said, Strengthen me, O Lord God of Israel, this day.

And she smote twice upon his neck with all her might, and she took away his head from him.

(JUDITH, CHAPTER 13, *HOLY BIBLE*)

I'm in Patrick's car in Kiwanis Park. Snow quiets the whole outside, as though we're the only people left in the world. I've been out of the hospital for two weeks, maybe three. I feel older.

I'm breaking up with Patrick.

Why? he says.

You weren't there for me, I say. After I was raped.

It's hard to say the word: raped. Even now he doesn't want to hear it. I'm afraid he thinks I went looking for it. His silence accuses.

Maybe he just doesn't know what to do with it. He doesn't want to know things like this happen. Like I'm a cat who's been hit by a car, dragging my mangled hind legs into the kitchen, hideous and bloody.

We can still be friends, I tell him.

He laughs, a short, surprised sound. No, he says. We can't.

I have other dreams. I know I'm supposed to be a wife, and that thought comes with a certain ecstasy, as in the ecstatic visions of Catholic saints, but I imagine other futures for myself. There's no conflict in my teen mind between surrender to a man and an artistic life. I've been on stage since I was six, danced *The Nutcracker*, acted in *West Side Story*, played violin in the orchestra for *Nutcracker* a year later. I wrote plays in fifth grade that were performed for the whole school and wrote sonnets for Patrick, entire letters in iambic pentameter. My ambitions are grandiose. Friends sign my yearbook and write: *Can't wait to see your name in lights!!!*

I drop out of Provo High. I think I'm going to live openly now, claim my fucked-up life. An honest apostate. I go to Mountain View High for a while. I keep sluffing school. I drop out of Mountain View.

I have to come clean with Dad. Enough sneaking around. I've been leading a double life. I say double life to my friends like I'm a secret agent. Secretary by day, crimefighter by night. But yes, sure. I put on my paper hat and work at Der Wienerschnitzel during the day, driving the Bobcat, now bald-tired and finicky. Pick up my lessons at the strivingly named Master Academy, home study school for dropouts. Come home and do homework, watch TV. At night I go into my room and put on my nightgown. Kiss Mom and Dad good night. Get into bed and pretend to fall asleep. After the house goes quiet, I get up, put on my clothes, sneak out my bedroom window, and spend the night at my new boyfriend's house.

Otherwise known as the Party House. A shifting collection of metalheads live here; Boris has his own room in the basement. Everybody's hair is long. Boris has corkscrew curls that fly when he plays guitar. He plays guitar better than anyone I've ever met, better than a teenage boy should, and he loves me. He loves me the way Dad loves Mom.

At the Party House, my flattop is petted, good luck like the Buddha's belly. At sixteen, I am the youngest one allowed into the circle. Alice is the benevolent mom of the whole crowd. No more than twenty-six, she's the owner of the house and so carries a certain maturity. A bottle of Southern Comfort passes around the living room where Boris plucks at his unplugged guitar, and I read *Catch-22* aloud for Stewart, a particle physicist who also happens to be illiterate. He might be severely dyslexic.

Stewart's car was the first place I smoked pot. Sitting on Boris's lap, I laughed when I realized I was high and they didn't know it, laughed harder when I realized my laughing might tip them off.

I'm hungry, I announced. Stewart cracked up.

Denny's, said Stewart.

Denny's! echoed Boris.

I jumped, having forgotten he was there. Quiet Boris, it seems, gets even quieter when he's high. That night in Stewart's car, he made himself so invisible I forgot I was sitting on his lap.

A family. I have a family here at the Party House. Easy and accepting.

Maybe, I say to my friend Anika, if I tell my parents my whole truth, maybe if I act like an adult by coming clean, then they'll treat me as an adult. I say this as we're leaving Planned Parenthood with my first pack of contraceptives. After the rape my stomach was chill lead until the results of the pregnancy test came back negative. This at least I can control. Anika and I drive together to Salt Lake City. I forge my mother's signature and get the pill, and then I tell Boris I want to have sex on purpose.

We are in his room in the basement of the Party House. Someone had started to stencil fleur-de-lis around the moldings, but they stopped partway through. The last few fleur-de-lis show the color underneath; whoever it was ran out of paint.

Are you sure? he says.

I'm sure, I say.

I want to cry that he asked me if I was sure, and I'm embarrassed, it feels like I have to ask all over again. But his face opens into a nervous smile. He wants it, too.

He lets me lead. He's on his back and I lean down to kiss him. I straddle his narrow hips and lower myself by stutter-steps until my pelvis meets his. I hold there, looking at him. I lean forward onto his chest. Face in his curls, my eyes leak slow tears. We begin to move against each other, but I can't make our rhythms sync up. His hips rabbit against me but it's too fast, I can't keep up. I don't know how people do this, I'm unbearably clumsy.

He's half-Mormon. His dad is Mormon, his mom isn't. He smokes cigarettes and acts like the church isn't especially relevant to him. I envy him his apparent freedom. I want my parents to see me for who I am. I want them to accept me the way nineteen-year-old Boris and all the metalheads wandering through the Party House do. Seems simple enough as I hold in a lungful, pass the joint to a sleepy-eyed man with stringy blond hair.

One night my timing's off in sneaking out. Boris is waiting outside in his truck. I can see his headlights through the scrub oak. I don't wait for the hall light to switch off. I climb out and jump into the truck, coast silently down the hill. It's quiet at the Party House, just the two of us. We get high and watch *Repo Man* in his basement.

I climb in my bedroom window the next morning, put on my night-gown. Unlock my door and there is Dad, waiting.

I knocked on your door last night to remind you of an appointment, says Dad. Where have you been?

Oh. There it is. The whole edifice collapsing. Years later I'll see the Seat-tle Kingdome implode in massive clouds of opaque dust, and I'll remember this. Now's my chance. I've been talking big about wanting to be treated like an adult, so let's do it. Let's give all of us a chance.

I tell Dad I'm on the pill.

We're sitting at the dining table, a dark wooden slab from Mexico, big enough for the whole family to sit together. Dad's at one end. I'm in the corner seat, facing him. His blue eyes go wet.

I'm glad, he says quietly, you're taking precautions.

Tears crawl down his cheeks. Dad cries every year when we watch *It's A Wonderful Life*, but I've never faced him when he cries.

I made Dad cry.

I'm going to have to tell your mother, he says.

Now my insides seize up. No no no, I think. I take his hand. He's already getting up. Gives my hand an abstracted squeeze, disappears down the hall.

I will describe the sound that came from the bedroom as operatic, but the truth is, I won't remember. Nothing. I can see Dad's blue eyes tearing up as we talk at the table, but I cannot retrieve Mom in this moment. Maybe there is no sound at all. Mom gulps in and smothers all sounds in the house, even the push of blood in my ears, silenced.

Depression is anger turned inward, Mom has been wishing to obliterate herself for years. She could not protect me when I was seven and molested by my cousin. She could not protect me at twelve, when I was assaulted at BYU. I had my first pelvic exam in the dark, in secret, because I did not believe she could weather the knowledge that I'd been raped. I thought I was ready now, I thought the worst was over. But learning I had sex on purpose is too much for her; her self-hatred is now unsheathed and shining. I can see it in her face, but I can't retrieve the sound that goes with it.

Now Father and Mother are in the living room, Dad jolted into performance of discipline, too late, too late. He slaps me across the face, then muscles me over his knee and spanks me. We're all in this trailer-trash opera now, all of us wailing and sobbing. We catch our breath, look away from each other.

Dad says they need to talk. I am to wait in my room. I do not wait. I get dressed and start walking out the back door through the mudroom. I am blind and trying to escape. I'm on the back steps when I feel my father's hand heavy on the back of my neck. He pulls as though he is going to lift me by my scruff like a kitten, and I clatter back inside.

We've been talking about Heritage School, says Dad.

(Mom appears to be past words. Her face is ... what. Immobile. A wall. Terrible to look at. I can't look.)

Heritage School is a reform school, a particular kind of bad teenager school. Mom used to work for its sister school, Provo Canyon. Provo Canyon is for boys, Heritage for girls. Beefy guys kidnap you from your house in the middle of the night, drag you off to Heritage. The ACLU perpetually had several suits going against both schools for abuse.

Okay, I say now to my parents. What's the alternative?

Well, says Dad. You could marry him.

All right, I say. I'll marry him.

We have a station wagon. It's not ours, we have never owned a station wagon. It belongs to my brother's wife's family; we're just car-sitting it. It's the logical choice for today's excursion. We load into the car. Bench seats means I can sit in front, between my parents. Escorted like a child bride with a pissant dowry.

As we drive to the Party House, Mom speaks.

You're not a murderer, she says.

What she means is, you're right next door to one. What she means is, she has failed utterly. What she means is, really, I might as well be a murderer. What she means is, I've killed her.

I know her this well. I know everything she means.

All the times I thought I was protecting her, I was protecting myself from her.

We arrive at the Party House. The lead singer from Boris's band is on the front lawn. He watches us pull up, and through the windshield, I see him mouth two words:

Oh shit.

He disappears into the house. A few minutes, then Boris appears, looking rumpled, his long curls still shaped to the pillow. Well, we had been up all night, getting high and watching *Repo Man*.

He gets into the back seat. Mom and Dad sit iron-faced on either side of me. I look into the rearview mirror. His eyes are open, wide, on me.

Dad keeps his hands on the wheel and proposes to my boyfriend.

Yes, says Boris. He looks at me in the rearview mirror. Now he's crying. Teen love! You can say Dad has Statutory hanging over his head all you want, but this is love. As far as we know how to do it. Nineteen and sixteen, true love. Boris is sincere; since we've been dating, he's been showing up on my front porch all scrubbed up, did his best to wash away his cigarette halo but all he managed was to smell like cigarettes and soap. He believes he is ready to make a marriage.

I am not. But my options have narrowed to this. If it takes hitching a ride on a boy's heels, I'll do it and get free of my tarpit of a home, divorce sweet Boris in a headspin. Soon to be a sixteen-year-old divorcée and just watch the blaze I'll leave in my wake.

And so from the back seat of a borrowed station wagon, Boris says *Yes*, and like that, we're engaged. Dad lays out the plan. We cannot get married until Boris can show he's ready to support me. I don't know what picture my parents are carrying in their heads. Dad didn't want to know, didn't want to look as I grew and wanted and lopsided my way into personhood. He doesn't know who I am, and Mom sees only sin in my face, so they are acting out this silly throwback spectacle, they will fumble the two of us into some *Leave It to Beaver* teen playhouse where Hubby brings home the bacon and I'm surely knocked up by seventeen. It's all over now—they failed and their last-ditch gift is stuffing me into a parody of domestic idyll.

~

He has to support me. No job as of yet, but we add that to the agenda. Every other Sunday he will come to our house for a financial planning meeting with Dad. This is as grim as you picture it, Boris is shined up in his button-down shirt and good jeans tight around his skinny hips, hair corralled into a ponytail—it kills me, it's the best he can do. He and Dad sit at a corner of the dining room table while I chew my cuticles and look off into space. I am there as a reminder: this is why we're here. I have no other role. They are totting up numbers that seem to have no connection to me.

I have a job. Der Wienerschnitzel, okay, but it isn't nothing. Correction: I *had* a job. Dad escorts me to the red doghouse and waits in the car while I quit. Dad's strong-arming Boris into a job while I'm forced to quit mine, because, again, it has to be the guy who's the breadwinner in this parental fantasy. I am under house arrest anyway, can't be trusted to go to work on my own. Anika calls and I hear the other extension pick up when I do. Mom and Dad want me to know they're listening in. I keep my conversations short. Marty, who took me to his junior prom at a rival high school, is worried enough to come to my door. Dad tells me there is someone to see me, reminds me that all I am allowed to say is that I can't talk to him.

Years later, Marty will tell me that while he is waiting for me on the porch, he notices a slim glass brace propped diagonally in my window. Dad placed it there. If I open the window, he'll hear it shatter. This isn't something you can buy off the shelf. It must have been a piece leftover from one of his sculptures. From art to child escape detection system.

I don't open the window. For over a month, I don't open my window.

The stool I used to climb out the window, the same stool Robert Fagg stood on to kiss me after delivering the paper, is gone.

Dad escorts me to Master Academy to pick up my lessons, take tests.

Alternating Sundays, I go to Boris's parents' house. Where Sundays at my house are sterile, Sundays at the Eastmans' are alive. Boris's father is a Braziliophile: his first wife—Boris's mom—is from Brazil, and so is Boris's stepmom, who now folds me into her bosom for a giant hug. The house is full of uncles and aunts and cousins three times removed. His stepmom makes a feast of feijoada and artichokes steamed tender. His father plays Brazilian songs on his guitar and translates the lyrics for me, all of them desperately tragic love songs sung to easy, swingy little tunes.

My parents call ahead to extract promises that we won't be alone together for even a moment, and Boris's father cheerfully agrees, then just as cheerfully edges out of the library so we can kiss.

I almost think if I get these people in the bargain, it might be worth staying married to Boris for a while.

Aside from this, I rattle around the house. I read. I do homework. I Think About What I've Done.

This is my glorious engagement.

A little over a month passes, and it's time to see the therapist. I've only seen him a few times since my release from the hospital, but he seems humane. A reasonable sort of guy. He looks like Gene Siskel, tall, thin, big head. He asks how things have been since we last met. I laugh so hard I can't stay in the chair. I'm kneeling on the floor and my hands are covering my face and I say, I'm engaged! I'm engaged!

He squats in front of me with a paper cup of water.

I find it terribly, horribly sad that I can't remember this therapist's name. He is forever Gene Siskel, and when the real Gene Siskel died, I cried like it had been this therapist, his name slid down a fathomless hole in my memory.

I take the paper cup and sit where I am on the floor, my back against the chair. He sits on the floor facing me. I tell him the whole story.

Condoms are also good, he says. Prevent diseases and easier on your body.

Yes, well, I say. With the pill, I'm in control.

He nods.

He has a whiteboard in his office. I'm staring at it. In my head is a picture of this whiteboard. Heritage School is written on it, there's a red circle around it. Marriage is in another circle. This is only my memory. I do not believe he actually wrote these things on his whiteboard, but all things are possible.

You don't need to go to Heritage, says Gene Siskel.

Yes, I say. A red line is drawn through the Heritage circle.

That place is . . . I'm not convinced it's such a good place, he says.

I nod.

You're too young to get married, he says.

Yuh, I say. I'll get divorced as soon as I can.

I see D-I-V-O-R-C-E in red letters on the whiteboard.

Divorced at sixteen? he says.

I'll be out of the house, I say.

What if you could just be out of the house, without getting married? he says.

I cover my face again.

Do you want me to talk to your parents? he says.

I hold very still. Is it possible? I nod. He gets up from the floor, flips his tie from his shoulder back into place, offers me a hand up. Dad is waiting just outside. Gene Siskel calls him in, and I wait.

After a while, Dad comes out and sits next to me.

Is this what you want? Do you want to leave?

I nod, looking at the floor.

Maybe you can stay with your aunt and uncle in California, he says. Let's go home. I'll talk to your mom. We'll make some calls.

It's that easy. I've been beating against the walls of the home like a cage, searching out the rules on emancipation for minors, want out, want out. But even I know that's too extreme. No judge would take me away. No abuse here. A big, loose, loving religious family.

And then my parents just open their hands and let me go. They give me up.

There is no breakup with Boris. My parents decide I'm to leave and I'm packed by the end of the week. I'm not allowed to see him to say goodbye. I just go.

~

When I was a kid, we had a great-hearted dog, Moby Dog. When my brothers were too much I'd sit on the back steps and lean against Moby, his right dogbrow raised in dignified sympathy.

We went to Paris and he ran away. I miss him still, want to put my arm around his shoulders and feel his easy forgiveness. I miss him but I don't wish him back. He's free of his chain, our tight backyard. Even now I picture him swimming the Atlantic in his search for us, grand dog adventures in his wake.

When I am in college I'll learn he never ran away at all. Our cousin had been staying in the house while we were gone, and she told my parents that a neighbor kid shot him where he was chained in our backyard. He never made himself free, not until his soul was freed from earth.

Families are forever is a church motto. When they die, the righteous are housed with all their family in the Celestial Kingdom. Husband, wife/wives, children. My sins are a wound to my father, I am putting myself out of his reach. When we die, I will have to live in a lower kingdom, a distant neighborhood. I will not be permitted to take a single step into the Celestial Kingdom. I will only be allowed occasional visits from Mom and Dad, like a child of divorced parents.

The Aughts

BACK WHEN I WAS A teenager, Gene Siskel had said the pill was hard on the body. Was I on it too long, did it fuck up my hormonal balance so completely I sprung a leak? My sins visited on me twenty years later, broke open in a river of blood.

Mom's funeral was Monday. On Tuesday, Gabe and I fly back to San Francisco. My friend Meg picks us up at the airport. Her mother died when she was in college. We are driving into San Francisco in the dark, and Meg talks about seeing her mother's body. She was alone with it, for just a few minutes. She says she put her hands on the body, found one spot that wasn't completely cold, just behind an ear. She kept her fingers on that spot as long as she could.

This cracks me. I start crying in the car, quietly, tears running down my face in the dark.

Mom, Mom, Mom.

A last failure. I didn't touch her body. I can't remember the last time I touched her. It's not like those stories where you regret that you didn't say I love you. We said *love* every time we talked. It's that I can't remember the last time: Not the last time we spoke. Not the last time we touched. Body of my body, and I refused to touch her in the end.

Thursday I am not allowed to eat anything but clear broth.

Friday, surgery.

1985

HOME HAD BEEN A HAND pressed against my chest. Already I feel released, I can take in a full breath. I'm driving my '64 VW Bug to California. California! Sun on my left arm, wind a ruckus through the open window.

The car begins to cough, seize up. I stop in St. George but I do not go to my grandparents' house. Mom will not have told them about the shame I've brought to the family, and I have no explanation for my trip, alone, sixteen.

The car is vapor-locking, I know what to do. Buy wooden clothespins at a gas station on the ragged outskirts of town, fasten them along the fuel line. Enough to get me to the top of the long hill into Las Vegas. Here, the Bug gives it up. I coast as far as possible, then have to pull over. I call my aunt in Las Vegas from a payphone. My uncle comes and hitches the VW to his car with a towrope. I have to ride the brakes all the way to Vegas. It's exhausting, I've been holding my teeth closed for miles.

Can't even make it to California on my own.

From my aunt's house, I call home. My brother answers the phone.

Hey, did you know Robert Fagg? he asks.

Yeah, sure I do, I say. Just saw him before leaving town.

I'll never know why Mom and Dad let me ride with Robert a few days before I left. Maybe they were finally tired of it all.

Robert's dead, says my brother.

What? I say. I plug my other ear with my finger.

He's dead, says my brother. He was riding his motorcycle on the grass in Kiwanis Park.

Kiwanis Park is at the bottom of our hill, where Apple Avenue T's out. You have to walk through Kiwanis Park to get to Wasatch Elementary. When I was twelve I walked through Kiwanis from school to meet Robert in an abandoned house on Ash Avenue, where I took off my shirt and ran across the room so he could watch my nonexistent breasts bounce. My whole body blushed and I curved my shoulders in, giggling, put my T-shirt back on.

Later that year he was kidnapped to Provo Canyon boys' school. Now eighteen, he'd turned into a man with wide shoulders. Took me for a ride on his motorcycle and we skipped rocks together. This was only days ago, so close I can still feel his breath at my hairline as he hugs me goodbye.

The cops started after him, my brother is saying.

For riding his motorcycle on the grass.

High-speed chase through the neighborhood, he says.

He was going over 80 miles an hour when he hit a speed bump.

All I can see now is Robert Fagg on his back in the street. The grass was bruised and so Robert had to die. Robert Fagg bouncing high into the air like a cartoon character. Robert Fagg spread all over Birch Lane, torn open throat to crotch, blood boiling out with his last awful breaths.

Robert Fagg is dead and I am going to California.

It's night when I arrive in Glendora. My aunt shows me around the house. My bedroom with a window to the front lawn, the street; my uncle's studio in the garden out back, forbidden to me; the large kitchen with an island in the center.

You can keep your food on this shelf, she says.

I realize she is telling me that their food is off-limits. My new freedom comes with conditions:

1. I must pay for my own food, school supplies, everything. My aunt invites me to join them for dinner the first night. After that, I'm only to eat with them when invited. This will happen rarely.
2. I must renovate my bedroom. I will tear up the carpet to reveal sixties-era green linoleum. I will patch holes in the walls and paint.
3. I must scrub the bathroom, one of my jobs when I was at home.
4. I must dust porcelain shepherdesses, commemorative plates, and glass shelves in my aunt's shop, and vacuum on my hands and knees. She will not trust me with the upright—understandable, considering my history with vacuum cleaners and art—handing me instead the furniture attachment.
5. I must attend seminary. This is Dad's stipulation. He hopes my faith can be salvaged. I will spend class breaks on Smoker's Hill with my cigarettes and new friends, then roll down the slope to seminary still smelling of smoke. Just often enough to get a passing grade.

It's worth it, it's all worth it. My aunt and uncle are on their way to Israel. They leave before I've been there a week. They'll return, then go to New York, return, leave, leave. No parents no jailers nobody waiting up to catch me out.

I am cast in a local dinner theater production of *South Pacific*. I will take home leftovers from the buffet after each performance, enough to keep me well fed.

For the first read-through, we sit in a circle. David, one of the seamen, looks brightly across at me. He's brown-skinned and keeps the whole cast laughing, his jokes will become our collective in-jokes. After the second read-through he asks me to his apartment. He kisses me as we undress and fall into his messy bachelor bed. I sleep all night spooned inside the curve of his body. In the morning I find my purse where his dog dragged it, the strap chewed right through.

She's jealous, she wants all the attention, says David.

I am shining from his attention all day at my new job. I face the shelves at a health food store, shift jars of organic peanut butter, make vegetarian sandwiches at the deli counter, and I'm thinking of David, his body wrapped around mine as we slept. We go back to his apartment twice more. I put my purse in his dresser drawer and he fucks me where I stand, bent over his dresser. It's over quick, then he pulls me into bed next to him.

By the time we're in dress rehearsals, he's stopped calling me. At the cast party we all knock out several boxes of cheap wine and his high-wattage smile is back, he puts an arm around my shoulders and breathes on my neck. My body floods with relief, he still wants me. Drunk he drives us to his place, drunk he undresses me, drunk he passes out. I don't know yet that drunk attention is a lie. I don't know yet that I'm as bored with him as he is with me. In the morning we're rumpled and smelling of bed, he's chatty as he drives me home, and we never see each other again. The play is over and so are we.

Alan in *Joseph and the Amazing Technicolor Dreamcoat* is white and unhandsome but he has an aura of authority and nobody challenges it. He's married, has a daughter my age, a younger son. He takes me to dinner at a white-tablecloth restaurant. I get steak and he orders wine for both of us; I look older than sixteen and anyway nobody questions him. When his wife is away he brings me into the shower with him, washes me like I'm his child. His washcloth misses nothing: behind my ears, in the folds between my legs, between my buttocks. He writes a sonnet comparing me to a diamond.

I turn seventeen and the cast presents me with a chocolate cupcake, a single candle to blow out. They all applaud. I have a rush of feeling, I belong with these people.

Alan is Mormon. Glendora is lousy with Mormons. We're sitting in his car after rehearsal. I'm curious: he still goes to church, still seems to believe. How does he square belief with adultery? To me there is a hard line: I am a sinner, therefore I do not belong in the church. I go to church meetings (rarely, just enough) because Dad demands it but I can't claim belief. I don't understand how Alan isn't destroyed by cognitive dissonance.

He tells me prohibitions against such petty sins are for lesser men.

How do you know you're one of the exceptions, one of the great men? I say.

Little men don't have the courage, he says. He's sliding his hand up the inside of my thigh. I don't stop him, but his touch is suddenly irritating.

An ouroboros, the fact of his behavior justifies the behavior.

When I break up with him, he writes his best poem yet, bitter and lit.

Tod is an Egyptian surfer who works the sound board. He takes me to the beach. I smoke too much pot and get too much sun and I'm holding onto sand while he carves an elegant line along the face of a wave, his long body so beautiful I have to look away to undazzle my eyes. He gets jealous when I talk too long to another guy backstage. After the show we park under the freeway and I listen to him yell.

Just take me home, I say.

He starts up the car and drives fast, throws us angrily around corners, I'm knocked against the door.

I'll leave you right here. Right here by the side of the road, he says.

Fine, I say. I'll walk.

I have no idea where we are. It's dark and all I can see is grass on the shoulder of the highway.

Tsh, he says. He drives me home.

A man wants me and I think it means love, when we are naked together it *is* love, I love him in that moment. And then we get dressed and it falls away.

I flirt, but not because I want to have sex. I don't even know how to have an orgasm yet, sex is how I show I'm sincere. I flirt chasing the light in a man's face. If I land my eyes on his for a full two seconds, I can see myself transform there. I become special, and he becomes lighter and happier than he was two seconds before. This is my gift: I can make a man happy, and it's too easy. Why pine for the unattainable guy when the one who returns my electrical signal is right here, when I can encourage him? *Good job,* I say with my face. *You're doing great at being a man.*

That charge, the change in a man's face, will light me up all my life, no matter how many times it is the exact wrong thing to do, the wrong man to cheer.

Anyway it's there in the scriptures. My job is to make my husband happy, cheer him up, lighten his day. And if you are to be good at it, you have to start practicing early.

But you also have to be careful. Spread that gift too widely and it loses value.

Hi Dad, I say into the phone.

Hi Sweetie. How are you doing?

I'm writing for the school newspaper, I say.

Oh, that's wonderful, says Dad. He sounds tired.

I want him to believe I'm a good person even if I'm not a good Mormon. I want his approval.

Dad, I'm on the yearbook committee, in the school play, I write for the school paper. Look Dad. All I needed was to be free, Dad.

Monday I walk into work an hour late. I have no excuse. The manager is at the cash register. Her skin looks like a damp paper towel. She spends her weekends partying in Palm Springs. Monday mornings she locks herself in the back room and I bring her dry toast until she's able to deal with people. This morning she had to open the store by herself, hungover and pissed.

You're fired, she says. Go home.

You can't fire me, I quit! I say.

She half-smiles and shakes her head.

Yeah, I don't believe me either.

Until now I'd been mostly living on tuna sandwiches from the health food store's deli. My food runs out quick.

I'm walking to school through the neighborhood. Every other house, it seems, has a lemon tree in the yard. Lemons weigh down branches, lie in the grass. Nobody will miss a few. I pick a lemon and bring it to my nose. It smells sunny and sweet. I peel it like an orange as I walk, pull it into sections, pop one into my mouth. My whole face clenches, neck muscles pull my mouth into a grimace. The second section goes down easier.

Lemons instead of blueberries.

I can't tell Dad I've failed. I've failed both of them, Mom and Dad. One more disappointment and all three of us will break under the weight of shame. I lost my job but I will succeed in keeping this from them, at least this. Dad can't afford to send me money anyway.

A few days of lemons and my taste buds burn dead. I'm peeling another lemon when a sudden sob comes out of me. I'm on the sidewalk and just one tear slides down my nose. I look around in quiet panic. Wide suburban streets, lush lemon trees, nobody on the sidewalk but me. Alone alone alone.

A set designer asks me out and I tell him straight up that it has to be dinner, and I get to take home all the leftovers. This becomes my requirement for any date. I eat all I possibly can at an all-you-can-eat buffet, I eat until it hurts. When I babysit I lay waste to the fridge. I'll finally get a regular babysitting gig, all the food I can eat.

For more than ten years, on every date, at every buffet, I'll eat like I'm starving.

I'm in Utah for Christmas. Mom is propped up in bed. I stand at the far end of the bedroom. I have an armful of stories for her, fresh from California, but her face is brittle. She wants me to see the violence I've done, the aftermath in her body.

One week and then it's time to go back to California. Dad finds a posting on the ride board at BYU, and John is sitting in our living room. Dad must approve him before he'll let me spend thirteen hours in a car with a stranger. While I'm under Dad's roof, I'm still his responsibility. John leans his elbows on his knees, tells Dad about his English degree from BYU, his wife back in LA, his mother here. They stand and shake hands. John looks at Dad's painting over the couch. It's abstract, burlap on canvas, oranges and blacks and yellows.

It's called *Conversation*, says Dad.

Oh, says John. I see it. Two figures.

Exactly, says Dad. They're Relief Society ladies.

They look monstrous. One has her mouth gaping open. John shows the edge of a smile.

See? says Dad. She has the light of the Gospel in her mouth.

They crack up, John's cheeks pinking.

We've been in the car five hours, John and me. His near-stutter is already familiar to me. It would be wrong to say dear about his voice, about him. Bright. We're driving slowly down the Vegas Strip and my brain is lit up, blinking in counterpoint to the casino lights as we pass.

I think I remember how to get there, says John.

We are turning down smaller streets, behind casinos, doubling back.

There! he says.

A tiny pizza place, red door two steps down from the street.

So I'm climbing back in my bedroom window, I say, and there's Dad.

The pizza's almost gone. It's a good story, a hilarious story, how I ended up leaving home.

Oh no! says John.

I know! I say. So I think, Okay, the jig's up. Might as well come clean, right? So I tell him I'm on the pill.

John's laugh busts out around his bite of pizza, he has to cover his mouth until he recovers.

The sky is paling when we get to my street. He stops in front of my aunt and uncle's house. We sit and look out through the windshield.

We're going to hang out, right? I say. You and your wife and me.

I really imagine this. The three of us, around a fireplace maybe. Cheese and sparkling cider. Talking and playing boardgames into the night. I will love his wife as much as I love him.

I'd like that, he says.

I get out with my bag, watch him drive away. I feel clean and wide open, the sun's edge just appearing above the houses.

John calls.

There's a new Kurosawa movie, he says. *Ran*. At this little art house in Venice. Would you like to see it? You and a friend.

My friend cancels at the last minute. It's just John and me in his car.

Listen, uh. He blushes. My wife and I are getting a divorce, he says.

I don't want to think what it means that I feel a trill in my chest at these words.

Ran isn't playing. We see another movie, one we know nothing about. *Brazil*. We sit beside each other, knees close, hands almost touching. I can feel the heat from his hand, feel molecules shifting at the surface of his skin, and by the time Robert De Niro appears onscreen, we're holding hands.

We're holding hands and my heart thunders through my body, feet to scalp.

Oh! I think. This is how it's supposed to be.

John's love is redemption. He forgives all my depredations (I tell him everything, even the photographer who invited his roommate to join us in bed. I would have done it, I would have, but the roommate had an appointment). If John can forgive me, so can Heavenly Father.

So can Mom.

Maybe there's a place for me in the church after all.

So I ask him to marry me. We love each other. We have never been naked together but we tremble along the borders of sin, he flicks his tongue under my bra, so close to my nipple I want to crack open, two more millimeters, one, please, please. But we stop ourselves, every time.

Marriage is necessary. He would have asked me eventually, but I am seventeen and I am bold and I tell myself I'm free of gender roles and I like the story this way better. I ask him, and he says *Yes*.

But not until you're eighteen, he says. My wife was seventeen when I married her. I want to do it right this time.

My English teacher shakes her head at me.

You're too young to give up your freedom, she says. You have so much life ahead of you.

Being married isn't the same as being dead, I say.

To me, the adventure begins with him, he opens my world.

John takes me out for sushi. I've never had it before. I'm unsure about the whole idea but I'm game and the salmon fills my mouth like a kiss.

I have something I need to tell you, he says. He blushes.

I've been married before, he says. Before my last wife.

A light stutter as he speaks.

They had two kids together. When she remarried, her new husband adopted the children. He has no contact with them now.

We've talked about the babies we'll have together. Nick and Molly, we've already named them. He had danced an imaginary baby on his lap, blushing and laughing. I wonder at this, how he could let these beings slip out of his life so completely. But he has forgiven so much in me. I cannot begin to hold this against him. I cover his hand with mine, kiss his mouth as it trembles.

John moves me and my duffel bag back to Provo in the springtime, the prodigal daughter returned.

Mom is charmed. John sits on the edge of the bed with his self-deprecating laugh, and she opens her arms to him for a hug.

We'll have to kill the fatted calf, she says, laughing.

I am on the right side of that hard line now, the side of the righteous.

Mom and Dad are thrilled when I tell them I want a patriarchal blessing. It's the custom to fast beforehand. I manage two days without food, go with my grumbling tummy to the patriarch's house. He lives in our neighborhood, halfway down Apple Avenue. During work hours he's an orthodontist. He's set aside a room in his basement for patriarchal blessings, where he will receive prophecy that is tailored specifically to me. He places his hands heavy on my head.

You will marry a righteous man, he says. You will have many sons who will be upright before the Lord.

I feel Something during the blessing. I feel my heart beat harder. The Spirit is supposed to feel like a burning in the bosom. This must be a burning. The Spirit, or a burning wish for the Spirit.

Mom takes me shopping for a wedding dress, snaps pictures as I try on one, then another, another. Froths of lace and ruffles and sequins. A far remove from my black-on-black clothes, heavy eyeliner. My hair is growing out now, permed and Sun-Inned to brass.

John moves out of the apartment he shared with his ex-wife, rents a place in Pasadena. I take a quick trip there to see what will be our apartment after we're married. There's an arthouse movie theater down the street. There are trees and hardwood floors and our own pots and pans and an archway between the kitchen and living room and I love it, my heart is light and tumbled.

No furniture yet. We sit on the floor, a pot of steamed broccoli between us, we are picking it out with our fingers.

There was, he says. You have to know. There was another wife.

This one between the first and the last. But it was only six weeks, only an elopement. All three of his wives were under eighteen when he married them. I will be different. I am inspired by my own generosity, my capacity to forgive. I go home to Provo, ready to plan our wedding. We run up his long-distance bill but we don't care, it's love, it's all for love.

On the phone he tells me he's thinking of moving back to Provo.

You should go to BYU, he says. You're a faculty brat, he says. Half tuition is a big deal. Family nearby will be good for both of us, he says.

The Pasadena apartment with its archways, the trees outside, slipping away from me. Provo closes in around my head.

The Prophet is head of the church and the husband is head of the family. You receive your orders and you accept.

Are you sure? I say.

It's best, he says.

Mom lost her temper with Dad once. I was a kid. She threw a sandwich at him. None of us can remember what it was all about. I have sandwich-thrower inside me but now I'm practicing obedience. Patience.

John gives up the apartment he'd rented only a month before and moves back to Provo. He takes me shopping, filling out my closet with silk blouses and wool skirts—he's trying to clean me up. I put on an outfit and model it for him and he blushes hard, stutters *Wow* and *Wow* again. I feel wrong in these clothes, but for him I do my best. Still, I throw out the floppy bows that are supposed to go at my neck, find excuses to never never wear the black silk pants, top the pleated skirt with a man's oversized shirt.

I've finished my high school career at Master Academy, and I'm asked to speak at graduation. Black sheep makes good. This is my moment. I wear a white dress he helped me choose.

After the ceremony, John comes back to my parents' house with me. He leans forward on the couch, elbows on knees, like the first time he sat here for Dad's inspection.

Listen, he says. I've been seeing another girl.

He puts his lips together in his nervous manner.

Well, woman, actually, he says. She's my age.

And it's over. He hadn't bought an engagement ring yet, no ring to return. It's just done. He walks out of the house and he's gone.

I am stunned. Like a beetle flipped suddenly on its back, I'm waving my little legs vaguely in the air. I'm back in my parents' house in Provo, graduated high school, no fiancé, no clue what comes next. For him I'd thrown away the scholarship applications I'd gotten from Bryn Mawr and Northwestern and now it's too late for anywhere else, my grades were rotten anyway. My only hope to get into BYU is the ACT, and I'd missed all the official sessions and prep classes too as I skipped from school to school, had thought I wouldn't live through high school anyway, and then I was getting married and college was an afterthought, but now college is what comes next. I shut myself in my room for a week. I let clothes pile up around me and curl on the floor of my closet and read letters from old boyfriends again and again.

And then I have to come out and get on with it.

Mom hates the way my voice changes when I talk to a man on the phone, the softening, the caretaking. She doesn't know I use the same voice with her. But when I was with John it was all okay, disapproval wiped from my scorecard.

It is simultaneously expected for a woman to arrange her life around a man's needs, and shameful for her to do so. Maybe it's only shameful if the man isn't the woman's husband, or husband-to-be.

When I was twelve, I learned enough guitar to play "Delta Dawn," and I sang it in a country sob. The worst fate imaginable, a woman jilted, a woman without a husband, without status, without validation. Invalid. Delta Dawn and Miss Havisham and me, cautionary tales.

But I don't sink to Havisham-level self-pity for long. I'm barely a woman as it is. I got into BYU thanks to a late session of the ACT, and here I am, husband candidates as plentiful as candy. It is only later, when I am older, that I will be tempted to wear my heartbreak like an ancient wedding dress.

I'm a BYU student. We call it BYZoo, I am a Zoobie, back on the wheel like my brothers, my sister. I falter in my Mormonishness, date Boris again for a time. We try mightily to keep our hands off each other but give in and run to the drugstore for a condom late one night; I confess to the Bishop, take my lumps, lather, rinse, repeat. I break up with Boris and fall for someone else.

Today I am cuddled up with Mom on the bed. We have gotten closer since the John debacle, my misery linked me belly to belly with hers. She calls John The Sociopath, welcomes everyone I fall for with a Mom embrace, even Boris. Today we're in a giddy mood. Our heads lean against each other and I've propped one foot on my knee. Mom starts lightly tickling my foot with a capped pen, she drags it in long loops.

Draw for real, I say.

She takes off the cap, I shift to give her better access, and now she settles in with concentration. She draws a web that begins on the sole of my foot, grows and nets my whole foot, ankle. I'm ticklish, but she finds the right pressure. Mom can draw too—we sometimes forget she was an art minor in college. I like her cartoonish web. She pulls one strand up my ankle and calf, and near my knee she draws a charming spider, Charlottesque, almost maternal, benevolent. Mom and I are both afraid of spiders, so she makes a spider who can't be feared.

We admire her creation together.

I never should have named you Amie, she says.

You're Caitlin, she says.

Amie is the Pleaser, I say.

Exactly, she says.

I understand her. I mean I'm way ahead of her. I never much liked my name. Amie is the flirt, the chameleon, the one who changed her voice to mollify whatever man I loved, Amie is everything that was corrupt and flimsy in me. This moment I am on the lip of my old self and molding the new. I can become Caitlin and make it official.

Change your name, says Mom.

And so I do.

Amie means *friend* in French. Not a terrible thing, surely. But my identity has been too fluid, adapting to whoever is in front of me in the moment, *Ton amie, Ton amie, Ton amie.*

Caitlin is a derivative of Catherine. Meaning? *Pure.* The next week I find a name dictionary at the BYU library, read out the meaning to her, and she beams. Sure, why not, not just in the sense of sexual purity, in the sense of being purified by repentance. It's more than that. Mom lifts her chin and looks at me, her black eyes sharp.

You are strong, she says.

Pure as in undiluted. *Pure* as in full strength. *Pure* as in *Do not mess with me.*

I considered myself an apostate at sixteen because I didn't feel welcome in the church, and under the influence of Patrick. Now, I've come back into the fold under the charm of another man, although this isn't the story I tell. Like before, I make it out to be all my decision, all of a piece with my original rejection of Mormon hypocrisy, where now I announce that I understand: men are fallible, the gospel is not. Maybe I never stopped believing in the Mormon god; I just believed I didn't belong.

I say I won't be swayed by the failings of humans, but still—inside I know I was led here by my heart that wants so loudly to be loved.

The summer that Mom and Dad lived in New York City, before they were married, Dad took her to a play about Caitlin Thomas, the poet Dylan Thomas' wife.

After the play, Mom wrote the name in her journal: *Caitlin. Caitlyn. Kaitlin.*

She meant to give the name to her second daughter, but there were boys and miscarriages and boys and then she was done. I was never supposed to be born. *Caitlin* forgotten until I was eighteen. I don't know it, but people are beginning to name their infant girls Caitlin. There are no Caitlins in my acquaintance, but twenty years from now there will be a profusion of Caitlin/Caitlyn/Kaitlins, all of them twenty years younger than me.

The second time Mom named me, she named me after a woman known best as a wife.

I am in the bishop's office with my latest ex-fiancé.

Word from the highest levels of the church is that any righteous man can have a successful marriage with any righteous woman. Already there is a tendency to marry the first person you become infatuated with after you come of age. BYU coeds have always referred coyly to their MRS degree. But now it's hopped up. There are jokes about young men fresh home from their missions who will walk up to a stranger on campus and announce:

It has been revealed to me that you are to be my wife!

Which is not so far from reality.

These were the perfect conditions for my third engagement. And then I break it off. He demands a last meeting with the bishop. The bishop's office is a cramped room on campus. We're wedged tight between dark shelves. I'd spent the holidays in the ex-fiancé's parents' house in Saskatchewan, too cold to go outside, crowded in with board games, books, mismatched dishes, piles of dirty clothes in his bedroom. I want air. I want wide road.

The ex-fiancé compares me to Rachel in the bible.

Jacob worked for seven years and got Leah, he says. And then he worked another seven years to get Rachel.

Are you saying that you are willing to wait as long as it takes, asks the bishop.

But, I say. I'm not going to change my mind.

Yes, says the ex-fiancé. That's what I'm saying. As long as it takes.

With a convert's fervor, my ex-fiancé condescended to forgive me for all the men I'd fucked. (I didn't use the word *fuck*. I said I slept with them. Like children in pajamas, dreaming together.)

Forgiveness isn't what I'm after.

There is still a living animal of want in me for my ex-fiancé, his wide chest and square hands. But as he talks I feel the shackles clank around my wrists. Want flips to revulsion. I want the bishop to say something. He's the adult here. He needs to tell him to respect my decision. But he won't. He's egging him on.

I want to break down the walls of this office. Bust out of all of it. School, church, Utah, my own self. All of it.

Once, a bird got into the house. It panicked, rammed itself into walls trying to get out. It smacked against white wall and left a smear of blue-black blood. It was terrible. We tried to herd it outside but we only upped its panic, drove it against walls, again and again. Splatters and wingstrokes of bird blood. In the end we just had to wait for it to stun itself, then gathered it in a towel and took it outside.

Mom tells me she thinks she might have been molested when she was a baby. We're standing in the kitchen and she says this suddenly, no lead-up. By a man, possibly a relative. A man with status in the church. A recovered memory, like the children who accused their parents of devil worship. She wants my pity, my sympathy.

I want to slam my fist into her face. How dare she forget her abandonment of me in my need. How dare she push into my space, play the victim.

Does she even remember what I told her?

I make a sympathetic sound. I want to tear at her skin but I hold still.

Maybe it's true, and she is only trying to connect. Not performance, but a simple statement of what happens to girls. Or maybe Mom is searching for an explanation. A story that says why she is so broken.

I can't look at her.

One of the few women in the bible to have a name, Sarah got two. Sarai until she was past childbearing age, Sarah after she bore a miraculous child. She gets two names but is still known first as a wife, a mother. Abraham's wife. Isaac's mother.

We forget she was also Abraham's sister.

It's a summer evening. I'm at the gas station, filling up my resurrected VW Bug. Friends painted a peace sign in white shoe polish on the back window, I've left it in place.

Somebody says my name. At the next pump is Julie. She was my MIA teacher when I was fourteen. She has multiple sclerosis. The passenger side door is open, and she leans her head back against the headrest to talk to me. This costs her some effort; she can't lift a hand, a foot, her head.

I squat to her level and put my face close to hers. Her voice, too, seems drained of volition.

Listen, she says.

I lean closer.

Get out. Get out of Utah. Promise me. You're the one who gets out.

I promise her. I need no convincing.

It will be the last time I see her. She will die a few months later. Her husband remarried within the year.

The Aughts

I WAKE IN A TWILIT hospital room. The doctor holds up her fingers to illustrate how tiny my womb was. The size of a peach pit, or a walnut.

Tiny, pink, and healthy, she says, shaking her head.

Nothing to explain the havoc it caused. I try to picture my insides now, without a womb. Nothing. The nurse puts a button in my hand. The button delivers morphine, but only after a certain amount of time has passed. Still, it gives me a feeling of control. Press the button. Press the button.

Sandpaper sheets and hospital smell and hospital food and the overcold hospital room. I'm told that once upon a time you would be kept until you had your first bowel movement after surgery, but I don't know how that ever happened with this food, white bread and cheese and lunchmeat. Now insurance companies want quick turnover, churn people out, open up a bed for someone else. Two nights is quite long enough for me. I fantasize about clean sheets at home. The long bedroom curtains I insisted on before the surgery. I see those curtains, embroidered with vines. Our heavy bookshelves, the cats, art on the walls, my own shower, wind chimes, I'm hungry for it all. Home.

1989

I am in London with my parents on another study abroad. This time I'm here as a teaching assistant, not just my father's daughter. But the university surely sees an advantage in the three of us sharing a flat.

We live close, brushing elbows to the bathroom and back. I sleep on the floor behind the couch, my bedroll and duffel bag hunkered down behind living room furniture.

I'm taking a bath. Water thunders in and I slide back into recline, plug the faucet with my big toe and feel water push and pound it around. I turn off the water and close my eyes to listen to the plunk, plunk, as water shifts around my body.

There's a crash. I hear it, feel it under the water. I sit still for a long moment. I can pretend I didn't hear. I can stay here and be in ignorance for another thirty minutes before the bath goes cold. It's probably just that something was dropped. I cup water in my hands and draw it up and over my face. Now I hear something else. Mom's voice, but changed. My heart sickens.

I get out and wrap a towel around me, open the bathroom door. Mom and Dad's bedroom is at the other end of the short hall, really barely a hall, just three steps long. Dad is standing outside the room, a kitchen towel in his hand. Broken glass spills out under the bedroom door, shining in the hall light. The carpet is wet, damp spot ticking larger, creeping to Dad's foot. Mom's voice is deep, unintelligible, on the other side of the door.

Your mother threw a pitcher. At the door, says Dad.

He lifts his eyes to me. He's telling me she didn't throw it at him, but he doesn't quite believe it.

Let me help, I say, but Dad holds up a hand.

Go back and finish your bath, he says.

I step backward as if his hand is pushing me in the chest from the other end of the hall.

I—, I say. Okay.

I back into the bathroom and close the door.

A few days before this her medications were stolen. Dad carried them in a flight bag. A whole flight bag to hold all the things she takes to keep her functioning. He set it down to take a picture and then it was gone.

Mom is in bed for days while Dad frantically calls doctors, pharmacists. Mom in bed, light off. We're half a floor below ground level. We can see people's hips and legs move past the window if we raise the blind, but Mom keeps it down, nothing but shoes in the slim gap under the blind.

Amie, says Mom, her voice climbing from lonely dark.

Hi Mom, I say. I sit on the bed beside her, brush her hair from her face. It's Caitlin now.

How's Boris, she says.

I broke up with Boris, Mom.

He's a sweet boy, she says. He loves you.

I know, Mom.

Amie? says Mom.

I take her hand.

Where's Boris?

He's at work, Mom.

Oh, I'm glad he found a job, says Mom.

Where's Boris? says Mom.

It's weeks before all of Mom's medications are refilled. She gets out of bed. She goes to church, joins us for student discussions. All the students are gathered in class and Mom stands up to speak. She starts out okay, but her sentences begin to bend and loop, she's talking about semiotics or no now the beauty of that sinuous curve between subject and verb or no wait she's threading a bright line between the quick-beating heart of a bird and you and me and Heavenly Father that great semiotician and here the golden thread leads to sunrise speckled with our blood and—.

I don't stop her. Dad doesn't stop her. She goes on and on and then sits back down. I hear the rustle of skirt over nylons as someone crosses or uncrosses her legs. We sit in padded quiet a long moment before anyone speaks.

Years later, at the study abroad reunion, the former students will be goggle-eyed that Mom was glitching. They all thought she was talking so far above their heads, they couldn't follow because they were too dim.

Mom goes to church and eats with us and she's not buried in her bed. I can almost see her eyes spinning in her skull but she is coherent for whole hours.

I'm fragmenting, says Mom.

I take her outside, hold her hand as we walk to the park, sit beside a stone fountain. I hope the sound of the water will calm her.

She asks me to take her wrist in my hand, place my fingers on her pulse.

She places her fingers on my pulse. She breathes heavily.

Wedding ceremonies in the Mormon temple feature the *patriarchal grip* between bride and groom at the altar. The index finger is placed upon the other's pulse.

I am not allowed to know this, as I haven't married in the Mormon temple. As far as Mormons are concerned, I haven't achieved full womanhood.

Mom is, sane or not, a Mormon mystic, moving just to the side and in the shadow of mainstream Mormonism.

We can't sit here, says Mom. There are demons in the fountain.

I take her hand to help her up, and we look for a demon-free place to sit.

~

There are hurricane-force winds in London. The front window in one of the student flats shatters inward; the girls come home to a carpet of glass and wind singing through their homework. Great old trees in Green Park are yanked up by their roots, left lying impotent on their sides. I walk home from school and feel a great shove of wind, grab hold of a lamppost before I'm pushed into traffic. Traffic is stopped, streets blocked off because slates are flying off roofs, half of London is on foot, and the sense of disaster brings British cheeriness to full strength.

Quite the weather, isn't it? say grinning strangers as we pass.

Mom and I are walking by a sidewalk café in a small alley when a hand of wind reaches behind us, picks up chairs and tables and stacks them in a messy pile against the wall. It happens double-quick, like an overcranked silent film. Mom starts to laugh, then covers her mouth and looks at me.

Did that really just happen? she says.

It did! I say, and we stand together, laughing, Mom's cheeks red. This outer chaos syncs up nicely with her inner storms and for a minute I think she feels less alone. Or maybe the wind is carrying her dangerously far from solid ground, and she has no choice but to enjoy the ride.

I get a flu that won't let go and Dad gives me a blessing. As Dad places his hands on my head, I feel Mom's hands join his, weighing me down. My neck stiffens. Her breathing gets noisy and obvious the way it does when I have to feel her pulse. While Dad gives the blessing, Mom murmurs words in a heavy stage whisper.

Heal, says Mom.

And Dad works the word into the blessing.

Strong, says Mom.

. . . bless her to be strong, prays Dad.

Mom's breathing is pushy and my eyes are shut and I'm split. The good Mormon me who is planning to go on a mission and wants to live in the light of the church is horrified. This is riding along the edge of blasphemy. The other part of me, as much my mother's daughter as the first, shines inside at how Mom's mania makes her bold. There was a time, early in the church, when women participated in priesthood rites like blessings. The place of women in Mormondom is rankling in the attic of my mind, and I love Mom for shoving against that ceiling. (She isn't sane, I remind myself.) I am embarrassed for her, and I'm terrified. This goes beyond eccentricity. It is the difference between apostasy and heresy. An apostate steps from a coherent belief system into a competing system of equal coherence (even if that system is non-belief, it's still coherent). Heresy plays within the narratives of the gospel, but rearranges the pieces until you are in danger of confusing God and Satan. Mom is dancing in a between place that is dangerous.

Her breathing strikes me as performative, a bid for attention.

Only a few years from now I will be on my kitchen floor, gasping in breath after breath, desperate for the man I'm with to see my suffering. Many years later, my own mind will betray me. I will wish for someone to place their fingers on my pulse, someone to quiet my breath.

Every guy I date is a wrestle. His job is to push for more; my job is to hold us back. I am not good at holding us back, but I lose respect for a guy who pushes.

I'm on a boyfriend's couch in London, our bodies braided together, hands under clothes. We met at church. He's from a northern industrial town, his accent with its rolled *r* charms me. He unbuttons my pants and I grab his wrist, hold his hand suspended above my body. I want to be naked. I want him naked. I want all of it, enough with all this childish base-stealing, but he says he wants to marry me and if we want to be married in the temple (we do, we say we do), we can't.

Come on, he says now. Just, let me. Let me.

He's ready to scuttle our wedding plans so he can get his fingers wet.

Maybe he knows I'm not wife material anyway. Not worth the effort of staying chaste.

If you believe, I say, why can't you wait?

~

My bishop in London has an issue with saliva management. His bottom lip is a shiny red and he has to slurp between words. It isn't his fault, but it's unnerving when I confess my sins. He leans on his desk, looking at me.

He touched you—where? he says.

Sluuurrrp.

I—he—I unstick my eyes from his wet lips, look at the wall. My breasts, I say.

Anywhere else?

Really? I think. This guy. I mean, bless his heart. Was probably savaged in school, with that fantastic overbite and lusciously polished bottom lip, but . . . bishop? This is the man who is supposed to be best suited to hearing intimate confessions. Okay.

I'm half-tempted to offer more lurid descriptions, just for the punker self I haven't left entirely behind. But I resist.

No, nowhere else, I say.

This is a lie, but nobody, not even Heavenly Father, could blame me.

Mom will tell us years later that she was having almost constant hallucinations. Anytime someone spoke to her, she waited for Dad or me to reply first; it was the only way she was able to know the person was real. This strikes me as all the more sickening than a blithe ignorance of your own madness. Mom knew she was crazy. This sharp awareness of her own sideways mental state kept her monstrously vigilant, and it wore her down, wore her like a suit of skin.

When I am nearly fifty, I will have to wrestle my own slippery mind, and I will remember.

Mom, I will want to say. *I get it. I'm sorry it took so long. I'm sorry.*

Mom goes back to Utah early, leaves Dad and me alone to shepherd the students through the last month of the study abroad.

Later I will learn that in Utah, she went to the hospital for electroshock. This was a decision she and Dad made together before she left. I am horrified.

Electroconvulsive treatments, says Dad, correcting me. It's much better than it used to be.

When we return to Utah she's still having the treatments. After every shock, her memory is fried. She looks at me with empty eyes. Some pieces of her memory will never return.

My friend Dominique says we have to accept the concept, if not the practice, of polygamy. She's right. Our faith requires it.

Anyway polygamy makes sense, she says.

Women are more nurturing than men, she says.

That could just as easily be an argument for polyandry, I think. A nurturing woman can make half a dozen men feel loved. Does a man really need three, four, five women to tell him he's handsome, smart, capable?

So much need.

I am on dangerous ground. In the Book of Mormon, the prophet Lehi dreams the Tree of Life. There is a narrow path leading to the Tree, an iron rod you can hold like a banister. Away from the path is darkness. Out there you are lost.

The path grows fainter for me every day. Less convincing. There's a whole world beyond that childish iron rod. The church espouses a belief in the eternal rightness of polygamy. Sure, it's a sin in this life. (Why a sin? Was it only so Utah could be a state? We joke about this but we do not talk about this.) But after we die, in the eternities, a man's marriage extends beyond his singular earthly wife to wives and wives.

Celestial Marriage.

I would be fine with polygamy, says Mom as we lean against her pillows. As long as the other wives are frigid, ugly, and hard workers, she says.

We laugh.

She can't know what will come after she dies. She can't see the woman Dad will marry. It will be right for Dad, his second wife alive with energy; he shouldn't be alone. We are all capable of loving more than one person. But Dad will advertise his Mormon-style afterlife polygamy. In heaven, in the Celestial Kingdom, he will be married to both of them. And so his new wife's engagement ring will bear three sapphires: one for him, one for her, and one for my dead mother.

In the eternities, Mom will have only him. Her identity sealed as my father's wife.

We believe in Heavenly Mother. More people in the church are talking about her now than when I was growing up.

Why don't we hear about her? I ask Mom.

Maybe there's more than one heavenly mother, she says.

Of course. Heaven is polygamous.

Maybe, says Mom, she is more powerful than we can know.

Even if Heavenly Father has multiple wives, only one of them is my heavenly mother. My belief frays, but maybe I'm missing something essential. Maybe Heavenly Mother exists. Maybe I can talk to her.

I begin to pray to Heavenly Mother. I give myself over to a last breath of faith, leave my doubts under the bed while I pray. She is perfect where Mom is broken. Maybe she exists. Maybe she sees me. Maybe she'll take me safe into her goddess bosom.

And then one of the Apostles stands behind the podium at General Conference, the yearly church-wide meeting where official pronouncements of the church are made and reified.

It has come to my attention, he says, that some Sisters in the church are praying to Heavenly Mother.

I am chilled that he somehow knows the content of my private prayers. But apparently I'm not alone.

This is a sin, he says.

In reaching for a divine Mother, I was apparently an apostate after all. (No, not an apostate. A heretic.)

There are good reasons to leave the church:

- Black men can't have the priesthood. And then the prophet had a revelation and—hallelujah!—they can.
- Wives of black men (overwhelmingly black women) matter less than other wives; they do not get to have the priesthood in their homes. And then they do.
- Native Americans are brown-skinned because of sin. Generations of righteousness will whiten the skin. And then it isn't, and it won't.
- Heavenly Mother exists, and isn't it wonderful. And then it's a sin to try to communicate with her.
- Being gay is a sin. And then being gay isn't a sin, but acting on your gayness is.
- None of these beliefs are fully repudiated, no acknowledgment of the violence rippling outward from each brutal stance. It is simply changed and so.
- Women can't have the priesthood, but this doesn't even belong on the list. Woman priests? Absurd on its face.

I move to Salt Lake City, share an apartment with a young man. I put on an orange polyester dress with a white apron to wait tables on the graveyard shift. It's an hour-long bus ride to Provo for classes. There's a bed in one of the bathrooms at the Harris Fine Arts center and I catch naps here between classes. My ears ring from sleeplessness and the top of my head buzzes from the Mini-Thins I take to stay awake.

You have rent? asks my roommate.

Give me a few days, I say. Please.

After work the next morning, I throw my tips at him, jump into my jeans, and rush off to school.

On my way home from school I stop at an ATM machine. I've never used one before. There's no money in my account, but I want to see for myself.

Words appear on the screen: *Hello Caitlin.*

It knows my name, I think. I start to cry, standing on the sidewalk.

Back at my apartment is a hand-drawn poster on my bedroom door. It's a cartoon of me in my waitress uniform, coffee pot in one hand. Glued to the poster is a one-dollar bill I'd tossed at my roommate that morning, the first of my tips.

These two moments shine deep into my center, and they are earthly. My roommate a non-Mormon. The ATM machine an unbeliever.

Maybe this world is enough.

It would be a lie to say I lose my faith for reasons. I don't tally up inconsistencies, I don't make *pro* and *con* columns and step out of faith when the *con* column weighs more. There are people who weigh reason against faith but I'm not one of them.

If I was born a lesbian, says Mom, I'd be fine with the rules. I just wouldn't have sex.

Really, I say. Mom. I know what the family libido is like.

(We can talk this way; since I was engaged to John it is allowed, this is how we talk.)

Can you seriously tell me, I say, that you would be able to do that, knowing you could never, ever have sex? That the whole idea of your desires is sinful? It's one thing, I say, to stay virginal until you get married. It's another to have no hope ever.

Oh, says Mom. I hadn't thought of it that way.

Appalling hubris: Create a goddess. Many goddesses, why not. And then forbid us to know Her, Them.

For a minute, on my knees and in the exploding black behind my eyelids, I believed. I tried. I willed myself to see Her.

And the church thought it could corral Her, could shrink Her from Goddess to Wife.

I don't know what I believe, but the strictures of Mormonism are closing in around me.

Don't tell me I have to be shut up in a marriage. If I am to be a sexual being it seems I must be married. Enough. I stepped toward a bigger life when I was sixteen and I can't shrink back to fit. Disentangle sex from sin and I see that knot was holding me back.

I am leaving an entire faith (let's be honest, let's strip all the arguments away) so I can be free of shame.

It's easy to say I'm breaking free. I will learn, one day I'll learn: freedom has to be chosen over and over again.

A story in the ringing of my ears, in my shaking hands, my sleeplessness. My second apostasy. A story written on the body, read from my body. Fingers and teeth and lips leave marks that are there always, written over by other fingers, other lips, but the palimpsest remains.

PART 3: THE WIFE LIFE

Unto woman he said, I will greatly multiply thy sorrow and thy conception; in sorrow shalt thou bring forth children; and thy desire shall be to thy husband, and he shall rule over thee.

GENESIS 3:16, *HOLY BIBLE (KJV)*

The Aughts

I AM TRYING TO REMEMBER the last time I saw Mom alive. I want my last memory of her to be something beautiful, but I can't pull up anything more recent than this: Gabe and I went to Utah, was it last year? Mom didn't leave the bedroom. I went back there to talk to her, to climb into bed beside her, but she was diagonal across the bed, there wasn't room for me. I perched on the edge. She was eating yogurt. It was laborious. All her concentration was on her spoon, getting it from bowl to mouth. She was in her Hawaiian muumuu, ankles crossed. One ankle printed with a long scar from a break twenty years before. She was on her side in bed in her muumuu and farting. The room full of her gas. She didn't say much. No room to hug her with spoon and bowl in the way, and it was difficult to know how aware she was, if she knew I was in the room with her. She was farting and frowning at her spoon.

No conversation. I don't know if we even touched.

Mom didn't have Alzheimer's. She didn't have anything that could be named and categorized that would explain why she found her spoon so difficult. Dad said she was often fine, fully lucid. Dad said she sometimes called him The Man Downstairs. Dad said one day she had convulsions. Dad said one day she was aphasic. Dad had been saying for years they'd been reducing her medications, but I don't know what this meant. I don't know if she was damaged by the medicine she was taking in the moment or by years of medicines or by a particular combination of medicine—or if the medicine helped in some way and her own body's chemicals were throwing such lightshows in her head that she couldn't focus on the outside world.

I feel a powerful need to talk to her. I can't remember if we talked after I scheduled the hysterectomy. I don't know if she knew I would never have babies.

1994

I AM LIVING WITH MY boyfriend Malcolm and his mother Peggy in Seattle.

Peggy is up early in the morning. I can hear her busy in the kitchen. Glass rings, pans clank. Her hair is gathered into seven little ponytails, eyes bright with an overcranked cheeriness I recognize. In London, Mom often woke me early, singing hymns in a piercing soprano as she bustled around the living room. Peggy has just been diagnosed with bipolar disorder, full-bloom manic. She is built differently from my mother. Where Mom carried a double awareness of the slippage between her reality and ours, Peggy is fully convinced of her rightness; she brings a hideous energy and fervor to every action. The first we knew of her psychotic break was when she lit up a cigarette on a trip home from Denver and was kicked off the plane. We got her home and she brought with her twenty-five Levi jackets with florid embroidery and rhinestone designs. We don't know where she got them, what she paid, if she paid. Certain she will get rich selling these, she claims a street corner in Seattle and harangues passers-by, the jackets in a pile beside her. This is what she tells us. She says she chained herself to the streetlight, or maybe it was the jackets she chained. She comes home with no jackets and no money.

We are at dinner with another couple, friends from Malcolm's MBA program. We're drinking.

I'm a kept woman, I say. It sounds hilariously old world to me. It's a lie, or rather a joke. If anything, Malcolm is a kept man, but I would never say so to him, never rub in my advantage as the wage earner, and anyway I'm only a waitress at a sports bar. I've left Utah behind, but I'm constructed of the limited characters available to women in Mormonism: fallen woman or wife. Now in Seattle I can play with my story, make fun of the identity of Kept Woman while wearing it, I can live in sin with a man and still be a good person.

The men tell dirty jokes. The other woman and I laugh, but not too much. I tell about the day Mom took me into the bedroom while Dad went off somewhere with the boys. She opened the encyclopedia on the bed, showed me anatomical drawings of the female reproductive system. Fallopian tubes and ovaries and eggs and sperm, and after it was over I still thought you could get pregnant by sleeping next to someone, that the sperm just went through the skin by osmosis when you were unconscious. Everyone laughs, except Malcolm.

In the car, he says, Don't talk about sex in front of friends.

Wait, I say. You can joke about licking pussy but I can't tell a sweet story?

It's disgusting, he says. His cheeks are turning red. When he works out, when he has a lot to drink, when he gets angry, he gets a raccoon mask of red around his eyes.

Malcolm was raised Mormon, like me, but now he is an atheist. Some ways of thinking are hard to kill.

Shame is alive in me, its eyes bright, it tells me he is right.

When I was sixteen and in the hospital, I was prescribed lithium. I took it for a while but stopped when I moved to California. This history is useful. Peggy refuses to see a doctor, so I see mine and ask for a new prescription for lithium. This is a terrible idea. It is a terrible, wrong idea, but we are sleep-deprived with her in the house and becoming scared. I dissolve the tablets into her morning coffee. No way to monitor dosage, no way to know how it sits in her blood. She tells us she feels electric shocks in her hands and feet. She holds her steaming cup of lithium and says:

I will never take lithium. Never!

Steaming cup of lithium is Malcolm's phrase. He repeats it to me, laughing. We're both laughing, our humor getting blacker by the moment.

I'm working long shifts at The Ram Café and Sports Bar, then on to performances of the one-woman play I've written. A play about Simone de Beauvoir, who wrote *The Second Sex* but did not consider herself a feminist. I say I am a humanist, not a feminist, never a feminist. Malcolm would never be interested in a feminist.

Malcolm is studying in his MBA program all day and into the evening. We lie in bed past exhaustion, both of us on our backs, waiting.

I set a fire, says Peggy from the dark beside our bed.

Malcolm is on his feet.

I'll burn up the bed, says Peggy.

I find a small fire on the back porch, contained in a dish. Malcolm finds one in the oven.

I burned myself, says Peggy. She shows an ugly burn on her arm.

Let's put that under cold water, I say.

No! She hugs her arm close to her chest, twists her upper body away from me.

Fires out, we try again to sleep. There is no lock on our bedroom door.

I'm calling social services tomorrow, says Malcolm in the dark beside me.

I'm at work when they come over. Malcolm tells how the social workers sat on the couch eating our leftover Halloween candy. He told them everything, and they shrugged. Nothing they can do. She has to be an immediate threat to herself or others before she can be committed. He pointed to the burn on her arm. Shrug.

She walked through the room, saying *Get me a gun, I'll shoot him in the head.* Shrug.

That's not a threat? he said.

Does she have a gun? said one of the social workers.

Shrug.

I come home from work one afternoon, and as I'm walking up the hill, I see a pile of things in the middle of the street. Peggy bustles out the door, throws an armful on the pile, hurries back inside. As I get closer I recognize individual objects in the pile. My things. My clothes. My books. White pages fly up from the pile, twirl in the wind, tumble down the street. My script. The only copy of the final draft of my play, carefully typed. I take off after the pages, running and tripping and bumbling down the street, hands reached out in front of me. I'm slapstick, I'm Monsieur Hulot, I'm ridiculous, a page teases just beyond my fingertips, then lifts and flutters away. I crumple three random pages in my hands, too buzzed with sleeplessness to cry.

I don't know if it's the next day, next week, or two weeks later. I get home from work. My stomach already in its dread knot as I approach our door. The living room carpet sparkles. It's layered with broken glass. The glass front of the grandfather clock is on the floor in three long, jagged pieces. Almost every glass in the house smashed and spread over the carpet. Peggy crunches from kitchen to living room, hair in pigtails, talking. She's rhyming. She's barefoot. There's no blood. She's walking barefoot on broken glass but there's no blood. She's cheerily talking in rhymes.

Her feet are bare!
How very rare.
Watch her smash
Every glass!

She is a strange beauty, her big blue eyes in their dark hollows, short pigtails trembling as she walks. She knows she's clever, knows she's riffing genius; she is exalted and humming with life.

I walk by her and into the bedroom. I close the door and wait for Malcolm to get home.

It's dark outside when he comes in. I tell him to close the door behind him. He sits down on the bed, I get up and lean against the door. My hands are shaking. I put them behind me.

I'm done, I say.

I tell him my plan. He nods. I light a cigarette, keeping my eyes on him. I hold out my right hand and rest the cherry of the cigarette on the back of my hand. I let it burn in. The pain goes deep into my meat. I let the cherry go dark where it sits.

Now, I say. Call the police. Call social services. Tell them she did this.

While he is on the phone, I go to the bathroom and run cold water over my hand. The burn will keep digging in for hours, all night. It will keep me tethered into the moment when I might want to let my mind wander elsewhere.

Keep her there, say the police. We will be there in an hour.

An hour shattered into towering seconds. She knows something's up. She was at the other end of the house when we made the call but she smells it on us when we come out of the bedroom. She picks up a long shard from the grandfather clock. It is the length of a small child. She holds it at her waist, swings in our direction. I am behind her at some point. I put my arms around her, trap her arms close to her sides. I don't know how we get the glass from her hands. Maybe she puts it down. That moment is gone. She's swinging that glass and then she's opening the door and we're wrestling it closed and then she's sitting on the couch and we are holding her. She squirms and we tighten our hold. We hold her. We hold her. She is fighting to get free and we will not let her free. The night yawns wide and opens beneath our feet and we hold her. We talk about our day. We are grimly holding on and I ask Malcolm about school today, ask who he met with, ask about our friends.

In some parallel universe, we are still holding her.

And then the police come. There is a social worker with them. They ask her questions. Who is the president, they ask. What day is it. What is the year. She gets some answers right. Mostly she doesn't pay attention to the questions. She's just talking. It seems okay, it seems better, and then they usher Malcolm and me into the bedroom and out in the living room she screams. There are six cops out there. She begins to scream, it's just the beginning. Six cops and one five-foot-two woman in her fifties. She screams like she's dying. She screams like skin is peeling from her skull. Six cops and she screams for twenty minutes before they get her out of the house.

I have done a terrible thing. I did this. And more. She's held for seventy-two hours and then there's a hearing. I sit on the stand in court and say I was taking a nap and she burned me with a cigarette. I say I wake to my hand burning and she says:

Is it hot/Is it not?

Which is a lie. Her rhymes were better than that. She gets on the stand and talks about bombs in the desert and D-Day. Her language is poetic. I picture a mushroom cloud blooming over the desert, I picture Mom watching the above-ground tests, Mom as a girl, Mom with her family, the whole community, all of them watching smoke unfurl across the wide Utah sky, cheerleaders' pom-poms glowing white against the dark of the Bomb.

Peggy is committed. We see her in the hospital and she says:

You have to get me out. It's all crazy people in here.

Little by little she calms. She is given medication. She is held for a month, and now when we see her we have real conversations. She gets out and stays in a group home a while. And then she's on her own, she meets a man and they set up a cozy home in a trailer on the Hood Canal. We stay with her on weekends and catch crabs and talk into the night and she says she remembers this time like she was watching a movie, like it wasn't happening to her.

We don't talk about the burn on my hand.

Malcolm agreed to my plan, but it was my plan. My execution. He didn't offer to burn himself. He failed to save us, so I had to be the hero. I was the one to pin her arms, I made her drop the vicious shard of glass. If I hadn't acted, we might still be swallowed in her madness. I want him to love me more because of this. I want him to be impressed that I can coolly burn my flesh. I didn't flinch. This experience bonds us. Or bonds me to him. I will stay with him for eight years, largely because this story links us. We are lovers but we are also siblings, holding hands in the dark woods. This is the story I tell myself.

There's another story, one I keep hidden from my conscious self: He should have stepped in. He should have found a way to save us. I am auditioning to be his wife, but he takes me for granted. I want him to see me as someone worth working for. I scarred myself, for him. He has done nothing for me.

~

Seattle is violently green, fertile and breathing. Mold grows on our windows in the night. I step outside to smoke and the chill air cuts into my bones. A lid of gray cloud lowers over the city in September, doesn't lift until May, June, July. When the sun is out my body opens up to take it in like a flower.

I do not believe in God, but I believe in Something; maybe only in all this riotous life.

We live in a rental house near Green Lake in Seattle, walking distance to the local bar. I am cleaning the sink because I smell mildew.

I don't smell anything, says Malcolm. You're imagining it.

Isn't that a sign of manic depression, says Malcolm.

Manic depression often shows up in your twenties, says Malcolm.

It is entirely possible that I am bipolar. Mom is inside me, she whispers from every cell in my body. But the way he says this makes a sick fear in my stomach. I am not my mother. I will not be like *that*. He says these things and he means to hurt and it works. I'm shaking while I scrub, but I laugh.

I read that women have a sharper sense of smell than men, I say.

That's bullshit, he says.

Oh, you know better? I say.

They don't know what they're talking about, he says.

My vision begins to black at the edges. I see the sink in the very center of my view. Nothing else.

So, I say. Trying to sound light, joking. My voice goes tight. So you know better than researchers who have devoted their lives to studying this one thing because, why? Because you know better?

Because it's bullshit, he says.

On the phone Mom asks, half-serious, when we're getting married. She disapproves of Malcolm but it will magically transform to approval if he makes an honest woman of me.

He has to get a job first, I say.

This isn't my requirement. It's his. We sit on the front steps of our apartment building, legs stretched out in rare sunlight. I ask him, casually, if we will ever get married. Outdated habit of thinking still alive, I think marriage will make me a valid woman. It will mean Malcolm loves me after all.

I want to be able to support you first, he says.

An echo of my parents when I was a teenager, forcing Boris and me into these gendered roles. Malcolm has to be the breadwinner before he can be a husband, before he can make me a wife.

Another night I tell him about the man who raped me when I went to his apartment for a party.

You shouldn't have gone there, he says.

Rage comes up in me fast. I can feel it rising from my feet upward. I fight it back and ask him for mercy.

Please, I say. Be on my side. He shouldn't have done that.

You can't just do what you want, he says.

So it's right if I can't go outside at night and you can?

It's reality. You need to get it in your head. You go outside, bad things happen to you. That's just how it is.

I'm feeling cornered. I am actually in the corner of the kitchen, my back against the lazy susan.

Are you saying I deserved it?

I'm saying you should know better, he shouts. That was a fucking dumb thing to do.

I start to scream. I cover my ears and scream. I don't want to hear his words anymore. I'm crouched in the corner of the kitchen and I'm screaming until I run out of breath. I have a thousand things I want to say, a thousand defenses, but they're all stuck inside my mouth. My speech has ground to a dead halt. I am sitting on the floor of the kitchen, my hands over my head, crying.

I don't know how we made up. I didn't leave him, not then.

~

I call my parents. Both Mom and Dad are on the phone.

Is it normal for passion to die? I say. I mean, you settle into a sort of placid love, still love, and respect, but no passion. Is that how it works?

This is what Malcolm tells me, so I'm asking them.

No! says Mom. She puts all her heart into the word.

When your mother walks into a room, says Dad.

We act like magnets on each other, says Mom.

We can't get enough of each other, says Dad.

Forty-five years and we can't keep our hands off each other, says Mom.

Malcolm and I make an art of our house. We've painted the kitchen a forest green with white trim. I paint the trim freehand, satisfied with the crisp line I make. The dining room a dark antique blue. We throw grand parties, the bar stocked to overflowing. All night long, guests arrive and leave in waves until it's a small diehard group, drinking until sunrise. Pancakes and mimosas, and finally the last guests creep out into particulate morning air.

We are Scott and Zelda, I tell myself.

I get a contract job at Microsoft. It's the early nineties, nobody has experience with this stuff, so why not. My first day on the job I ask if I can take a lunch break. My manager cocks his head at me.

You can hook up a margarita machine to your desk if you want, he says. Just get the work done.

I've stepped into a whole new idea of workplace. I get the work done. I code. I do graphic design. I bug-hunt. Plug me in almost anywhere, I can fit. I skip from contract to contract, my rate rising with each skip. Malcolm tells me I'm worth more.

You should be making ninety bucks an hour, he says. You shouldn't have accepted forty. You don't know how to negotiate.

Meanwhile, he sits at home in his boxers. He graduated from MBA school years ago. He plays video games. He goes to the bar in the evening.

Friday nights especially are sacrosanct. Every Friday night he must go out to drink with his friends. I don't say that Friday night shouldn't matter if he does the same thing every day of the week. He can hear me thinking it anyway.

One day I tell him:

You're a lousy housewife.

I say it like it's a joke. He doesn't take it as a joke. He goes to the kitchen and gets my dirty dish from the sink and drops it in my lap.

I didn't know you cared so much about being a good housewife, I say, then bite my tongue.

I am a rude bitch.

We are looking at family pictures and Malcolm points at my sister.

She's got great tits, he says. What went wrong with you?

He laughs.

Just kidding, he says.

You're cute in kind of a British way, he says. But you'll never be beautiful.

I took it for granted I'd grow up to look like my sister. Like Mom. Dark hair, perfect figure, long straight nose. I see now I messed up, got it wrong. Shorter than both of them, small-breasted, crooked teeth, blobby nose, hair medium-boring-brown. I fucked it up.

I like being the breadwinner. I am competent. I am strong. I tell myself this. I'm not like other women. I am the breadwinner and most of my friends are men and I drink beer with men and I laugh at their jokes.

Secretly, I think: I'm the head of the household.

Malcolm has strict ideas about what things should cost so I sit in the car at the grocery store and take the price tags off everything before I bring the groceries home.

I'm not the head of anything, not even myself.

~

Men on the street call me *Beautiful*. I think this means something. I go home
and tell Malcolm that the man at the grocery store called me Beautiful.

Men will say that to anyone, he says.

I keep it inside. I know he's wrong. I need to believe he's wrong.

I stop going to auditions. I stop writing. I work software hours. Sixty hours a
week, seventy. I feel flattened out, like all my biggest emotions are spent and
now it's just a long gray fog until I die. I am unrooted in my sense of self. I
can't measure reality anymore. We have friends but I am not allowed to talk
to them about my private life. I talk to my friend from college, Belle, for half
an hour, and he yells up the stairs:

Are you still on the phone? What are you talking about? Are you talking
about me?

Afterward he is silent, punishing. I understand I am not to talk to Belle
anymore. She is threatening. I don't know what is real. Maybe he's right.
Maybe Belle is threatening. She calls him Mr. 8-ball. As in behind the.

I have given all my reality over to him. There is no external reality anymore. There is only him.

We buy a house. The money is mine, but the title is in both our names. One that's
walking distance to the bar, because this is necessary. Every night after work, we
drink. They know us at the bar, the owners become friends. I don't know what
normal drinking is, nobody I knew growing up drank. I think this is what people
do. Like *Cheers*. You go to the bar every night after work and get drunk. Only my
body gets tired of it. I'm overweight and my stomach is bad. I shit black. I go to
the doctor and learn it's a bleeding ulcer. I name it my Microsoft ulcer and then
I have to go off coffee and alcohol and most food. Coffee and alcohol were how
I moved through the day. The withdrawal is weeks of sick headaches.

I can't drink so much anymore but he still goes to the bar every night. I've had surgery to fix my sinuses and my nose while they're at it. Maybe he'll like me better with my new nose. He is helping his friend from MBA school study when I have the surgery, so a friend picks me up at the hospital.

I'm home and recovering and he's at the bar. I wait. It's two o'clock and the bar is closed, and Malcolm isn't home. Three o'clock. Four o'clock. Five. I get up and walk outside. He's standing on the street corner at five in the morning in the dark, talking and laughing with his friends. I take him by the arm and yank him away. I do not say hello to his friends. In the kitchen I yell, kick the cupboards. My nose starts to bleed.

I sit on the floor, nose bleeding into my bare hands.

I am a caricature.

I let this happen. It slipped in by little bits and here I am, the nagging wife in the movie, dragging him home away from his friends. I don't want to be this person. I got myself here and this is not where I wanted to be.

Mom asks again when we are getting married. My mother was once a wise-cracking beauty queen. Everything around her said she would live a copy of her own mother's life. Marriage, kids. But her insides pulled away from domesticity, she was going to be a writer. And then she fell for my father. She believed his East Coast sophistication would free her. But after my sister was born, you could see death in her eyes. Already tethered. Already boxed in. And now she wants the same for me.

I want it too. I want him to propose. I think if he proposes, it will mean he wants me after all. I'm ashamed for wanting this. This woman I am con-structing does not indulge pink-roses, one-knee marriage proposal day-dreams. I picture marriage to an atheist as superior, smarter than a simple-minded Mormon marriage. I don't realize I'm mimicking my mother's naive hope: if I hitch myself to someone worldly, I can escape my mother's fate. My cognitive dissonance climbs to a high scream by our eighth Valentine's Day. He's been saying he wanted to wait to propose until he had a job, and now he has a job.

He'll ask me now. It's so clear. He likes me in trousers, so I wear my second-hand Jones New York suit. I make him dinner, light candles. I'm ready. We sit at the table, and he hands me a box.

Happy Valentine's, he says.

Inside is a silver necklace. Wide flat links carved into abstract floral shapes. I try it on and feel its cool weight. It is maybe the most beautiful thing I've ever owned. I kiss him thanks and go to the bathroom and lock the door and sit on the floor and sob. I am sobbing because he didn't ask me to marry him, sobbing harder because it matters to me, because I care, because I put so much wanting into a black hole.

My love for Malcolm shoves hard into my chest. His arrogance and cruelty are part of my longing. I am so anxious to be what he wants that I have no room to ask what I want. I've always thought this is how it works: you find someone and your love for them feels like drowning and you stay with them forever. The end.

I've been engaged three times. I collected marriage proposals like charms for a bracelet, sixteen so far: Mormon men are compulsive proposers. I've lived with Malcolm for eight years, and I'm crying on the bathroom floor because he didn't ask me to marry him. All these other men wanted me, but he doesn't.

With the ulcer comes a recurring fantasy that carries me into sleep. An enormous boil develops on my chin, the kind I used to get when I was a teenager. I stare into the mirror and squeeze. A homunculus emerges. A frightful, slimy little creature. It embodies everything ugly, clumsy, stupid in me. I set it free and with the creature out of my body, I begin to grow. I'm five foot ten, five-eleven, six feet tall. My hair turns dark and shampoo-commercial lustrous. My breasts grow, waist narrows, I am blindingly beautiful, I am brilliant, I am powerful.

When I wake I check my image in the mirror. Malcolm is right: I'm not beautiful. My face is swollen and gray, clothes too tight on my bloated body.

~

Our good friend Gabe works at Microsoft too, in a building not far from mine. We meet for lunch now and then. We go off-campus one day, to an Italian place he knows. Gabe is half Italian, half Portuguese. We talk easy. I look up at him over my pasta and his face flushes.

We go to our separate cars in the parking lot.

Ciao, Bella, he says.

My heart clicks in my throat.

I find an excuse to drop something by Gabe's apartment. He invites me in. We talk. We are awkward. We are both laughing at nothing. And then we kiss. I kiss him or he kisses me or one way or another, we're kissing.

One minute he's kissing me and the next he's on the other side of the room. He looks at me wide-eyed like I just slapped him. If I'm honest, his kiss isn't that great. It's unfamiliar. But the electricity is real.

Gabe and I have lunch again, an Indian place. He knows all the best places to eat. In the parking lot, he hugs me. The hug lasts longer than a friend hug.

We fit, he says.

We kiss again. And again. Malcolm leaves town and I go to Gabe's apartment in a little black dress. I made the decision. He answers the door and we're in each other's arms. His kisses taste good to me now, taste wonderful. He throws his head back, his eyes wide and dramatic. I've lived with chilly, Teutonic Malcolm eight years. This kind of demonstrative thing is a little embarrassing. But then Gabe picks me up and carries me to the bedroom and I tear the buttons from his shirt and he accidentally bumps my head against the door frame and we're both cracking up and I'm not embarrassed anymore.

Afterward I cry, hard.

I've broken something, I say.

He holds me.

Adulteress, I think. I am an adulteress.

Just once Gabe came to my house while Malcolm was out, and while he went down on me, I hallucinated Malcolm's face appearing on the stairs. I should have made Gabe stop what he was doing, but I didn't, I rushed through a faked orgasm, and maybe he felt me pull away, maybe he felt the beginning of a chill, the first slim question to come between us.

I start to see a therapist. Gabe and I tell each other we'll stop and we stop and then we start again and we tell each other we'll stop.

I tell Malcolm I'm having doubts. I tell him we have serious problems. Ever since he got a job I've been waiting for him to propose, the specter of Wife hanging over every conversation. Now I say this is not the time for a proposal. I tell him I'm seeing a therapist. I ask him to come with me, go to couples' counseling with me. He comes with me just once. Afterward he tells me he won't go again.

I'm afraid what I would learn, he says.

Malcolm takes me to dinner at a new French restaurant. The chef was a regular at our neighborhood bar before he had open heart surgery, quit drinking and lost fifty pounds. He gives us special attention. At the table, Malcolm pulls out a small velvet box. Inside is a gold ring with a diamond. He asks me to marry him.

Now? I say. You're asking me now?

I leave the table. In the bathroom I'm vibrating. I can't look at myself in the mirror. I don't know that what I'm feeling is anger. I don't know this is rage. My hands are on the sink and my mouth is wide open and no sound is coming out. I have to breathe deep and deeper and I don't know how long I'm here before I can go back out and sit down.

I hate gold. I hate diamonds. Malcolm knows this.

My therapist stops in the middle of a session.

Listen, she says. I need to talk to you as a woman. You need to know.

This is abuse, she says.

He's abusing you, she says.

Get out, she says.

Signs of Emotional Abuse (partial list):

- He isolates you, forbids you to talk to your friends, forbids you to talk to family, forbids you to talk about your relationship.
- He tells you your tits are too small, your nose wrong, your calves malformed, you load the dishwasher the wrong way, you cross the street too clumsily.
- He says you are imagining that smell, that the newspaper lies, that you can't understand politics, that you are hallucinating.
- He is your only trustworthy interpreter of reality.
- He tells you what to wear, where to work, what salary you should command, what you should pay for groceries.
- You are not beautiful, he says.
- I am the smartest person in any room, he says.

I take a vacation by myself. I fly into Salt Lake City and see my parents, pose for family pictures. In the pictures I am puffy but my face looks open. The slender tree we planted when I was a kid is ten feet tall, broad and leafy, but the branches are too high and too slim, it is not the climbing tree I imagined. Mom is in her Heavy phase, she is sunk into bed. She lifts her chin like she's trying to look at me over the top of a shelf. I tell her I'm not happy with Malcolm. I'm beside her in bed and holding her hand and she tells me she loves me.

I drive south to my grandparents' house. Neither of them can manage stairs anymore. Grandma sleeps in the little room off the dining room, the room that was my great-grandfather's until he died. Grandpa is on the couch in the dining room. They talk to each other through Grandma's open door.

She's turned her face to the wall, says my aunt. My aunt brings them lunch and dinner every day.

I don't think she'll last long, she says.

Grandma manages a couple of words for me. Grandpa dozes.

I leave flowers in a vase on the table and drive into the desert. The air feels new to me. I can stop at a roadside hamburger stand if I want, no Malcolm here to disapprove of the calories or the cost. I book a room in a B&B at a hot spring in Hurricane, near Zion National Park. I soak in the springs and watch the sun set over red rocks. It's too much. It scares me, how much I love being alone.

At night, in my room, I call Gabe. Not Malcolm.

I am falling through the structures I've built, playing House with Malcolm for eight years. I'm falling like Alice down the rabbit hole, I can't imagine what I'll find at the bottom. I know I have to go. I move out of the house but tell him it's just a separation, I just need to think.

People who separate to think, says a woman at work, almost never go back.

I want to argue with her. I want to tell her I'm not People. I just need to figure myself out, and then I'll go back. I keep my mouth shut. I ask him to write me letters. A thin hope; finally, he can show me how much he wants me. It's not too late. He writes one letter. Five pages detailing the diet he's on, the new feeder he got for the cat, gossip about his friends from MBA school. Not a word of love.

When I was first seeing Malcolm, an old friend of his said:

He has a pattern. He makes life impossible for the women who love him. He does hateful things to them, but he tells them he loves them. He torments them until they have to leave him, she said.

I'm different, I said. I won't leave him.

At night my head is full of all the disappointment that will ripple outward if I leave him for good. My family disapproved of Malcolm but they have finally accepted him, allow pictures of him into the family calendar. His mother has found her own stability, and Malcolm and I as a couple are part of it. We throw famous parties with a generous bar and food I make from scratch. It's not just Malcolm and me, it's everything we've made together.

Malcolm is an atheist who believes in aliens, but Mormonism prepared me to fit myself to him. In the absence of a god in heaven, I made him my god. I bent myself to his reality.

It's only now I've moved out that I see clearly: Malcolm never made himself my husband, but I was always his wife.

Malcolm's mother, Peggy, calls me at work.

I'm at your house, she says. The couch is gone. What's happening? Nobody talks to me.

I'm sorry, Peggy. I moved out, I say. I need to think for a while.

Oh, she says. Well. I hope you work it out.

She already knows where this goes. We don't work it out. I tell him I'm never coming back. He leaves the house when I come back to gather my things. I leave him the bed, the mid-century modern dining table, the dishes. I carry out my father's artwork and my clothing, my books. He will buy me out of the house and I will never speak with him again.

The Time Traveler's Wife, *The Bonesetter's Daughter*, *The French Lieutenant's Woman*. It's an old story, women given definition through the men beside them. Mormonism is only a highly concentrated version of America, not something Other. Even out here in the larger world, I am expected to be the dentist's wife, the artist's wife, the killer's wife: whoever I hook myself to stains me with his choices.

With no husband no boyfriend no partner, I am alone, I am free and terrible. Right now it is too much for me to bear.

1999

ALREADY I'M IN LOVE. ALREADY speeding down that road. It's too soon but the love is a rush, his love for me, his desire. I tell him I need time alone but he calls while out for a walk and confesses he's outside my apartment. It would be wrong to tell him not to come up. Instead I rush down the stairs and out on the street like a scene from a movie, I jump into his arms, I have never felt so wanted.

I call him Gabe after the Gabe in *Far from the Madding Crowd*. Gabe the quiet guy who loved her all along. Gabe the good guy. Gabe the happy ending.

I'm taking my daughter out for french fries, says Gabe.

His daughter from his first marriage; I've never met her.

Want to come with us? he says.

The girl is hiding behind her father's legs when I answer the door. I tip my head to look at her. She peeks out, one hand clutching his jeans.

Hi, I say. I wave my fingers at her.

I go to a monastery in Southern California. A single bed in a monk's cell. Dirt paths through the stations of the cross in the foothills of the Santa Ynez Mountains. Repelled by Mormonism, another religion looks exotic to me. Two quiet weeks among the monks will cleanse me, redeem me.

A decent interval before jumping feet first into a life with Gabe. I tell the monks I'll be in silence. I need to be alone with my own head. Only I can't stand my own head. I can't bear the loneliness. I read and I write letters to Gabe. Pages and pages every day. After eleven days in silence I'm jumping out of my skin. I pull aside a monk and tell him I need to talk.

It's okay, he says, laughing. It's not a contest.

I get a ride down the hill to the beach, call Gabe on my new cell phone. It's a terrific relief to talk to him, to feel tethered, wanted. His desire for me is irresistible.

My grandparents, Mom's parents, die. Grandma and Grandpa, both of them on the same day, Grandma on the very lip of turning a hundred. Grandma had slipped into a coma. I can picture it all.

Mother, called Grandpa from the sofabed.

Dear, he said.

She didn't reply. For seventy years she had replied every time he called. His heart tripped and shuddered and beat itself to death.

And then Grandma woke from her coma.

George, she said.

No reply. Mom tells us that Grandma knew he was dead. And so she turned over in bed, face to the wall, and stepped out of life.

Grandma was hard, Grandpa quiet, but they were soft on each other. Grandpa would pat her bottom as she moved past him in the kitchen. Her cheeks flushing, she swatted his hand away.

My family held them as the model of celestial marriage. In Mormonism, very few people can have their *Calling and election made sure*. This means your seat in first-class heaven is reserved before you even die. Prejudged and stamped on the forehead as near perfection as a human can be.

If anyone can have their calling and election made sure, said Mom, it would be them.

(I don't know that she'd forgiven her mother's angry curse hurled at Mom and her two sisters: *I hope you have three little girls just like you.*)

I felt Grandma's disappointment radiating outward every time I visited. No matter how carefully I stepped, she shook her head at me.

When I was fifteen, Grandma came to stay with us for a week. A friend stopped by to see me. After he left, Grandma wrinkled her lips at me.

Why can't you play with white boys, she said.

Mom shook her head when I told her.

Oh, yeah. That's Mom, she said.

Racism clearly not a barrier to heaven for Mormons.

I choose a plum-colored dress and fly to St. George for the funeral. In honor of their love story, black is entirely wrong. I am building a love story with Gabe, and if we are lucky it will end like this. I'm done resisting the pull. I want to be loved for sixty years. I want to be safe. I want to be seen, known, *wanted*.

I go back to the quiet of the B&B in Hurricane. This might be the last time I travel alone. Gabe isn't much for traveling. I can't forget my MIA teacher Julie at the gas station when I was a teenager.

Get out of Utah, she said.

I hear it now in my head: *Go.*

Back in Seattle is a man who loves me, who will never humiliate or box me in the way Malcolm did. That's worth more, worth everything.

I stop at the motel to pick up Mom and Dad for the funeral. Mom isn't ready yet. Sweat has wetted her curls to her face.

Peter, she says. I'm shaking.

He asks her what medications she's taken.

Look at my hands, she says, putting her hands in his.

Here, he says, and she opens her mouth like a baby bird for him to deposit a pill on her tongue.

She leans into him.

I don't know what I'd do without you, she says.

After the funeral, my siblings gather in the parking lot. We talk about Mom, about what we'll do if Dad dies before she does.

A brother says, Let's hope that doesn't happen.

The sick one always lives longest, says my sister, or maybe I'm the one to say it.

We all nod as though we have pronounced a universal truth. We have no answers. We only know Mom's up days are fewer, her down days longer; we know we see dimly inside the marriage, even the siblings who still live in Utah don't know what every day is like at home, only: Mom is not well, and not well in a steeper way than what we knew growing up. She's gathering speed, and any reach we might still have to help her is fast disappearing.

On his summertime birthday, Gabe brings me to the roof of his building. It's sunset. He opens a small box to show a simple titanium band. He looks at it, says, Oh! then turns it around.

The joke is, it's the same no matter which way you turn it.

He says, I wanted to ask you on my birthday in hopes of increasing my chances.

He slips the ring on my finger. We drink champagne and smash our glasses against the brick wall of the building next door, then cover our mouths and look down the canyon between buildings. Nobody seems to have noticed. We go inside to call our parents and Mom's voice rings with joy.

Oh, Honey! she says. I'm so happy for you.

I know she is. She's wanted this for more than ten years. I can feel her relieved exhale from here.

I serve Gabe the cake I made, three lopsided layers. I'd called his mom to learn his favorite. It's crowded with candles, and the top slopes alarmingly, all the candles clumped together into a near fire. He almost catches his hair in the whooshing flame as he leans in to blow them out.

This is my happy ending. This is what all the books and movies tell us. The woman is lost because she just hasn't found the right guy. She hooked up with the asshole but there was a good guy there all along, and once she sees him, once she makes her story about him, well, then she's got it right. Then it all works out.

Gabe really is the good guy. He loved me for years and never expected anything. The first to show up to help with a move, the last to leave. One of the parties Malcolm and I threw, someone brought a Polaroid camera. Gabe showed how you could play with the pictures as they developed. You take the handle of a fork and scrub the picture in a design that appears along with the photo. In a picture of me, he scrubbed a halo around my head, a cross in my hands instead of the fork I'm holding. Our Lady of 1996, he wrote on the bottom.

My brother Jonah picks Gabe and me up at the Oʻahu airport. Jonah's married now with a daughter, lives in a tiny house on the windward side of the island. He's driving us home and starts making Portagee jokes.

Gabe's half-Portuguese, I say.

Shhh, says Gabe. I wanted to hear the jokes. My mom collects them, he says.

Jonah puts us in the same room. No drama, no discussion. We're not married yet but I'm over thirty and we're engaged.

Mom and Dad are visiting, too. Dad's teaching a term at BYU-Hawaii. They're staying in the neighbor's house next door to my brother. It's my chance to introduce my fiancé to the family.

Mom is skinny. She had gall bladder surgery and a gastric bypass the year before, and her bones are fearfully thin. She's recovering from pneumonia, wears a Victoria's Secret nighʻtshirt all day. She's more tentative than ever, looks to Dad for cues. Gabe makes jokes and everyone laughs but Mom. She smiles uncertainly, holds her chin up, looking at us up-and-over, like she's holding her face out of water.

The second day, Mom is talking in dictionary definitions. I remember Peggy and her rhymes.

I was feeling frivolous, I say about a dress I bought.

Frivolous, says Mom. *Adjective. Not having any serious purpose or value.*

A chill creeps over me.

I like your Mom, says Gabe.

She's not usually like this, I want to say. But I don't know. I'm not living with her. I can't make any claim to what is usual.

Dad comes back from errands.

I went to the pharmacy, he says to Mom. They told me it's dangerous to take Ritalin with your antibiotics so soon after your pneumonia. They wouldn't refill it.

Mom takes in a sharp breath through her teeth.

Wait, wait, he says. I went to another doctor. And he gave me a refill.

He pulls pills out of his shirt pocket like a magician, like the pacifier he had in that same pocket when I was two and in the hospital after my tonsillectomy. Leda had thrown my pacifier away in frustration when I was screaming with tonsillitis. It's one of my earliest memories, light spilling through the doorway as Dad walked toward me in my hospital crib, my savior, his widening smile, a brand-new pacifier peeking from his pocket.

Mom lets out her breath, leans her forehead against his.

I'm taking care of you, Honey, he says. Just let me take care of you.

Gabe and I are standing waist-deep in turquoise ocean, my brother's house behind us.

This place is like another country, I say.

Only we already speak the language, says Gabe.

No work permits to worry about, I say.

Let's move here, I say.

Do you really think we can? he says.

He's never lived outside Washington state before. He's scared shitless.

Gabe and I have planned a trip to the Big Island.

Just before we leave to catch our flight, I go to say goodbye to Mom. She's in the bedroom. She's sitting up in bed, naked. I've never seen Mom naked except when stepping out of the shower. Married Mormons are supposed to wear their sacred garments all the time except when making love, bathing, or swimming. It's jarring. It's wrong. Her eyes don't focus on me. I hug her and feel her breasts loose against me and my heart goes cold.

At my brother's, I find Dad.

I'm worried about Mom, I say. She doesn't seem well.

I'll take care of her, says Dad. You go.

Every night on the Big Island, I cry in bed, Gabe's arms around me. I've failed my mother. She's in trouble and I left. Dad can only do so much; for long hours she is in the dark of her bed. I don't know what I would have done for her, but I left like everything was okay. I know she's not okay. I feel it in the hard knob of my stomach. Mom is sinking, and none of us know how to help her.

We get back to my brother's house five days later. It's evening when we arrive. Dad calls from the hospital.

You mother has overdosed, he says.

He asks me to go to her room, gather up all the medicine bottles and bring them to the ER. Gabe stays in the waiting room while I go in to meet Dad. I hand the box to the doctor. The doctor starts reading the labels. Each one prescribed by a different doctor. His expression shuffles through a handful of emotions.

She's taking all of this? he says. Maybe he's misunderstood.

Dad nods.

The doctor opens his mouth, closes it. He holds the box, touching labels with his free hand.

How long has she been taking this? he says, holding up a bottle.

Um, five years, says Dad.

The doctor stares, hand with the bottle stuck in the air.

You're not supposed to be on this for more than three days. It's for convulsions.

Yes, says Dad. She was having convulsions.

I look at Dad. I didn't know this.

Maybe five years ago? says Dad.

You—, says the doctor. And what about this? He pulls out another bottle.

Eleven years, I think.

That's, it's only supposed to be for a few weeks. And you shouldn't take this and this together. Or this. I don't—

He's young, the only doctor on duty in a tiny rural hospital. He takes in a quick breath, shakes his head.

We're going to have to pump her stomach, he says. I don't think you want to see this.

Dad and Gabe and I sit in the waiting room while the doctors work over Mom. There is no door between us and Mom. Just a half wall. We can see around it if we stand up and take two steps to the left. We stay where we are. There are terrible throat sounds on the other side of that wall. No other patients here, it has to be Mom.

Dad talks with me about the quality of the light coming in through the glass block windows, how it moves on the white tiles.

Do you see, says Dad, drawing a design in the air.

I see, I say. It's graceful.

The overdose didn't kill Mom, not then. Gabe and I had to fly home to Seattle the next day. When we left, Mom was in the hospital, where they would get her off all the meds. At last, I thought, we'd know what was underneath; she could start over. My first day back at work in Seattle, my brother calls to tell me that Dad had checked her out, took her home the next day. Dad's head swelled with memories of Mom in London after her meds were stolen. All he saw was terror. He told my brother that he didn't want us to mention the overdose to our siblings. I want to scream down the phone. That was Mom's chance, and Dad stole it, I tell my brother. I don't have the courage to say this to Dad. It's already too late, I think.

My parents feel there is some security, some hope for Mom inside all those pill bottles. But the medications will kill her, slowly and then all at once.

~

It takes us several months, but we do it, we move to Hawai'i. We have a small wedding after we've found jobs, a home. Mom and Dad come to the island for the wedding, but she is too sick to make it to the rehearsal dinner. We make do without the bride's parents then, a homemade spaghetti feast at our yellow house.

I don't see her until the day of the wedding. She walks in as I'm getting ready. She moves like she is made of glass. We hug for a long time.

I am marrying at last. Dad walks me down the grass, we hum Mendelssohn's wedding march quietly to each other as we go. Gabe and I set up chairs for all the parents, but they stand through the whole ceremony, even Mom. She stands to give her blessing. I am made whole for her, I am safe.

At the reception, she has to leave early. My whole family leaves with her. The reception is half-empty in her wake, the celebration cut off too soon.

Wife, I say to my new husband. Wife. I feel it on my tongue. I roll it in my mouth like chocolate, like a filthy word. Wife, I say, as I take his cock inside the word inside my mouth.

I'm married and back in the family fold. They can get over the fact that he isn't Mormon. He's funny, and he's married me, and that's really our biggest requirement. He fits. He's part of the family, and so am I.

Our yellow house is across the street from the beach. We wake up to the sound of a wild rooster crowing, go to sleep to the sound of the waves. We lie beside each other in bed and say:

We live in fucking paradise.

We take a picture of ourselves on our two-day honeymoon. The office where we both work wanted us back as soon as possible, product to ship. Gabe holds the camera as far as his arm will stretch, guesses at where to point it. This is before selfies, before smartphones. We won't know if it will come out until we get it back from the drugstore.

In the picture, we're flipping off the camera, joyfully. Fuck you, we're saying to our bosses. But we go back to work when they ask. Two weeks later we're laid off. Both of us out of work at once.

We have already begun to seal ourselves inside the walls of The Couple. Single friends drop quietly away; now we make Couple friends.

Gabe and I are unemployed, ten days after our wedding, ten days after the VP invited himself to our wedding, seven days after we cut our honeymoon short to come back to work. Unemployed in fucking paradise.

We're out of work but a good wife has no time for despair. No time for madness. She cannot allow herself to break. I've trained for it my whole life. But Gabe sinks. No interest even in sex. I plead with him. Sex is what keeps me going, I say. Please.

We make love with the windows open. I am noisy. We set the neighborhood dogs barking almost every time. Once, passersby on the sidewalk below stop to applaud. We lie beside each other on the bed, naked, laughing.

For years I'd set myself apart from other women. With Malcolm I held onto this idea: I'm not like other women. I'm better than silly, shallow, girly women. But now I begin to ease. I make friends with women. I am in no way superior. In fact, the women who have all along understood us as equally worthy humans are far ahead of me.

Gabe's daughter comes to visit us on the island. She's eight years old. He has a job interview, so I take her to the beach. We buy cheap board shorts and eat shave ice and when she slips her hand into mine, my heart rolls over.

Gabe hasn't found lasting work since we were first laid off. I am working but it's not enough, pay is low and jobs are few. The island welcomed us but now it closes itself off. We have lived in Hawai'i for the first three years of the new millennium, the years we call the aughts, but now we are ejected from Paradise.

2004

GABE HAS A JOB. So do I. Glory hallelujah. We have moved to San Francisco, a two-bedroom apartment five blocks up the hill from Golden Gate Park. After almost two years here I am beginning at last to feel settled, feel roots growing from my feet and into the ground. I've made it out of my twenties and no diagnosis of bipolar disorder. I am stable as a house. A set point of happy that I return to after every shock. Mom's curse hasn't seeped into me.

Dad tells me on the phone they are making progress. They got rid of their last doctor, but this one they trust. They are working, Dad says, to reduce her medications. It's been six years since her overdose. I don't know how much progress has been made. Mom isn't up to talking most times.

When she can talk, Mom says:

When are you having babies?

She wishes children on me, but her first child drowned inside her womb, his corpse floating inside her for months. And she went on to have six more, sinking herself deeper into the marriage bed with each one.

We're talking about it, I say.

She knows and I know what she means. A child will be the crown, the evidence, of my redemption story. My family loves me in spite of my apostasy. When I visit Utah, a brother may deliver his testimony as if it is a natural part of the conversation, but it has a special heat with me at the table. Tears-standing-in-the-eyes sincerity. The only answer I know to give is silence. Testimony may in fact be a regular part of dinner in Utah, I don't know. I've been away a long time. It isn't just the church. It's every story I know. To be a mother is to be Mary is to be whole is to be a purpose and a person and a power. A mother is a goddess in embryo, practice run for the great babymaking factory in the Celestial Kingdom. So I don't believe in that anymore, not literally, but this idea lives in our secular language too—parenting is godding is life is the creative principle at its electric, bawling source.

More than that, my body wants a baby. Baby hunger is a demon waking up inside me like Legion possessing the man in the country of the Gadarenes.

In San Francisco I am in hyperactive Good Woman mode. I cook. I clean. Our flat is charmingly eccentric, welcoming. A constant battle with clutter, with entropy, the falling-apartness of having and accumulating stuff. Warm colors. Dad's art on the walls. A poster from the ferry where Gabe and I danced in the new millennium, framed in Art Deco glory. Guests stay in the spare room and we walk to restaurants, to the park. Friends who drink too much stay over and wake to a good hangover breakfast. I am an apostate and so have to work harder to show I am good. When we visit my parents I fret over my clothes, my presentation. We maybe have sex more often or more enthusiastically than is quite proper for a married couple. Our neighbor either upstairs or downstairs leaves an unsigned note in our mail slot with just four ominous words: *I can hear you.*

But this sort of thing runs in the family. Children will round me out, make me a real adult, a full woman; in making a loving home for a child I will be shot fat with purpose. I can climb a level up from my parents, will be there for my child in a way they weren't. I promised myself I wouldn't forget the insults of childhood. For the sake of my own kid, I have not. I remember them all and will put my heart into making a safe bed for my children's tender roots, let them grow, let them become greater than me and my husband combined, let us rest in their shade.

Now is the time. I'm thirty-six years old. It has to be now.

I work on upper Fillmore Street in San Francisco. The wealth here is difficult for me to grasp. Five-hundred-dollar T-shirts, nine-hundred-dollar skirts in the stores. The women here are sleek, white, tanned, buffed, manicured. Every one carries an enormous diamond on her ring finger.

These are wives, I realize. Their entire job is being a wife, is staying beautiful for their rich husbands. It's a full-time job. You have to get your hair done, remove your unwanted hair, exercise your body, dress your body in luxe clothing, feed your body organic kale and flax seeds, get your nails done, teeth, breasts, and then start all over again with hair.

Even here, even in libertine San Francisco, there are women who are wives before they are anything else.

I judge these women. Some childish part of my brain is jealous of them. But I am a wife, too.

Of course children are part of the Mormon requirements. Birth control isn't exactly forbidden, but Mormons believe it is a primary responsibility to multiply. There are a finite number of souls in the waiting room of heaven, wanting to be born. They have chosen their parents.

If they've chosen you, and you fail to breed, you have deprived them of their choice.

And then, Armageddon can't begin until all the waiting souls have touched foot to earth. Multiply, or none of us will ever see the Celestial Kingdom.

These stories don't let go so easily. I have slipped the harness of belief but the training remains, my brain still twitching with expectation. My body amplifies it, openmouthed with an atavistic hunger. Baby, roars my body. Baby.

I've been taught since birth that my purpose in being alive has always been wife, then mother. The secular world amplifies this story: the happy ending of the rom-com a wedding, the Good Woman a mother; and the story lives in my body, deep beneath consciousness. To have a child is to fling a line forward into eternity. A belief in the future, in the only sense of forever left to me now.

And then I start to bleed.

~

My sense of time drifts. I am bleeding. After or maybe before the transfusion, another visit to the ER. This time they give me an emergency D & C, dilation and curettage. The cervix is dilated and the lining of the uterus is scraped out. It's common for miscarriages and early abortions, or after a birth when the placenta won't let go. There is a thin hope this will fix or at least slow the gush; the lining of my uterus is unusually thick. Nobody can tell me why I am bleeding, a thick lining as good an explanation as any. My arms are bruised black from multiple stabs, my veins have always been small and shy and the nurse slaps my arms to bring up a vein. I get an IV in the back of my hand this time.

They do the D & C in a room with a big picture window. I lie on the operating table with my knees up and look to my right to see San Francisco spread out below. The nurse gives me a drug that doesn't put me out, he says it's the best high ever, he says it's his favorite, he asks if I want more, and he's talked it up so much I do want more. I say, Yes, give me more.

I shouldn't have asked for more. Back in the room after surgery I start to vomit. I haven't been eating well lately and there isn't much there, but I throw it up and then I keep vomiting and nothing comes out but clearish green or greenish clear. One nurse holds my head and another holds a bedpan until there is nothing at all left to vomit, but my stomach keeps clenching, trying to eject itself from my body. The D & C was supposed to slow the bleeding and so I am only wearing a thick pad. I go to the bathroom. Blood gushes out of me fast. It runs down my leg and onto the floor and I slip in my own blood and I'm on the floor, crumpled against the door in a spreading pool of blood, and I think: *this idea of dignity is a fake, we're all getting older and if we live long enough someone will be changing our diapers, we are human and we are ridiculous and smelly and filthy and helpless alone.* I'm wedged between door and toilet, sitting in my blood, thinking this and crying and laughing at the awful comedy of it all. The door opens and I roll backward, try and fail to catch myself. The bathroom door opens outward. Of course. This is how bathrooms are built in hospitals, and in my mess of thoughts is unreasonable love for whoever designed this bathroom door to open outward. I don't know if this is the same nurse who was talking up the drugs but his strong arms are under mine and he lifts me into bed, cleaning and swaddling me like an obscene baby.

~

Months later, after the hysterectomy, Gabe helps me slowly up the steps to our flat. The sheets have not been washed. I've been dreaming about clean sheets, surely Gabe would have washed them, but he's a wreck, too. How long has it been, sick and then Mom and then Gabe tossing sweaty in the empty bed. I don't know how many days after the surgery before I am able to take a shower, can pull one leg after the other up and over the edge of the tub. The water thaws, softens me. I hold the place where my womb used to be and sob. I curl into a corner of the tub and open my mouth to scream, but I don't want Gabe to hear, don't want him to worry. I stop my mouth with my knee, my fist. I grieve the babies I will never bear, I grieve the woman I was. I grieve my mother, her half joke: When are you going to start having babies?

I am hysterical. *Hysteria: of the womb.* No more womb, no longer a real woman, but giving in to hysteria in the tub.

I feel amputated and guilty, sure that my sins have made me unworthy of motherhood.

I could float here in the soft dark of my bed forever. I turn to my side and my eyebrows draw together, like Mom's in a depressive phase, her disappointed look, that hard line zipped between her brows. I rearrange my face. I am not her. Look, I'm smiling. Look, my face does not shut off the way hers did, look at me laugh carefully around my stitches, I am not her.

I turn over in bed again and she opens her eyes. We are nose to nose in bed, my black eyes hers.

With practice maybe Gabe could become as good as Dad at bringing me dinner, keep the house going. Maybe he could take over the social obligations, write thank you notes, Christmas cards, remember birthdays. I don't actually do these things well or often, but I feel appropriately guilty about it. Those are the wife's duties, Gabe hasn't had the training. He doesn't even know they are required. The litter box becomes a scene of battle, or one of those Victorian stories, where the characters never say what they mean, not directly. He says he'll change the litter box daily if I remind him daily, but this is exhausting to me. I can't muster it. Friends come to visit and I'm sitting on the couch and the stench hits my face, I have to ask him to change it now, now. Still not supposed to lift anything, my stitches not healed, and so I ask.

It's safe here in sickness. Otherwise I don't know my purpose. It's the twenty-first century and still my purpose is tied to that reproductive organ that has been tossed out with the other medical waste, that peach pit–sized life-generator and why else do I exist. I've learned, thanks to the pink-trimmed HysterSisters, that there are different kinds of hysterectomies. I went for Total, which is not in fact total. It includes the cervix but not the ovaries, and so those babymaking hormones are still pumping away on their monthly cycle, brainlessly preparing my body to be a crèche, over and over. My cervix, gone. This allowed for a less invasive surgery, no visible scars, but I read that it can make sex feel different for the man. It's five weeks before we're cleared for sex again and when we do I ask him how I feel.

You feel like Caitlin, he says.

Of course I weep, we weep together.

I edge up to talking with Gabe about adopting, but he evades. How beautifully we avoid talking. The not-talking is embroidered, we talk all the time. We quote movie lines, we read to each other, we talk politics, we joke, I complain about work, but his job is slipping away, hours dwindling to nothing. We do not talk about his job search. We do not talk about adoption. It's clear, I can't mistake this not-talking for anything else: adoption is unimaginable to him. He was willing to half-close his eyes one day and make a baby with me, almost by accident. But to go to the effort and expense and paperwork—oh, nothing more exhausting and soul-sucking to him than paperwork—no.

For a long time after the hysterectomy, I am terrified that I will begin bleeding again. I bleed in my dreams, black, shining clots of blood passing out of me like living creatures. I will have these dreams for years.

I have been coasting, months given over to the crisp medical world. I recover slowly, then have another surgery for adhesions, a third for a Brobdingnagian ovarian cyst. Almost two years in and out of hospitals and doctor's offices. Being sick frees me from responsibility, from the heavy responsibility of keeping my husband and me afloat, of making his life okay, soothing his anxieties and keeping him safe. His job disappears entirely between my second and third surgeries. I am grateful my body took this decision—whether or not to have a child with Gabe—away from me. My body renders me blameless.

Except, of course, my brain is too well tuned to guilt to let such a fat plum go. I was so anxious to refuse responsibility that I broke my own body. The mind-body link is strong, and I will never know for sure. Did I do it to myself? Is this thinking just another way to claim responsibility, and guilt, for something I couldn't control?

I go back to work. Gabe spends his days at home, has to be rousted out on an evening, if he gets out at all. He isn't Malcolm, he is loving and hilarious and never unkind, but the Man on the Couch is familiar to me. I begin to wonder if he is my creation, my work of art. Man in Boxers. Gabe prefers the vaporizer to the bar, and this is another improvement but I am just tweaking the style of my creation: a kinder, gentler codependent.

Gabe is depressed. The realization soaks into me like dye into a shirt. I was fooled for a time, because it is hard for him to sleep. To me, depression = long hours in bed. Gabe barely sleeps.

My set point, I say, is happy. Mom was bipolar. Malcolm was depressed. Gabe is depressed. I seek out the romance of depression, but I am happy. I know how to be happy.

I keep getting sick. Different kinds of sick. I am paralleling my mother's trajectory, this constellation of diagnoses. No grand unified field theory of sickness, rather a looseness to us both, like whoever assembled us at the factory didn't quite get the parts flush. We are substandard material, still functioning but glitchy.

My blood sugar balances me on the edge of diabetes. My thyroid is low, sinuses still cranky even after surgery in my twenties. I have a sore throat for weeks, and when I open my mouth to speak, I throw up. My body is not subtle with its metaphors. I am growing isolated in the middle of my marriage and don't know how to span the gap between us. Speaking this aloud is dangerous.

I was a ballerina once but now I lose my balance unpredictably. I'm walking down the street and find I can't stay upright. Arms windmill like a cartoon, but nothing for it, I land on my face and eat sidewalk. My ears roar. A prelude to a dizzy spell that drives me horizontal, even the bed feels unstable, has to be the floor. I'll stay here for hours, eyes closed, until the spinning stops. I am diagnosed with Ménière's disease, an inner ear disorder. The unpredictable fall is called Crisis of Tumarkin. This cracks me up. Tumarkin, I think, as I get back to my feet.

Wifely qualities, self-test:

- Kindness   +8
- Caretaking   +7
- Sex: good at, taking joy in, saying yes to   +10
- Cooking   +7
- Sewing   -9
- Commitment   +4
- Hostessing   +2
- Social obligations: tracking of, execution of, grace in   -8
- Quiet   +1
- Supportiveness   +6
- Competence   +7
- Listening   +3
- Understanding   +5
- Modesty   -2
- Humility   0

- Thriftiness   +1
- Health   -8
- Childbearing   -10

~

Yael's *until* came when she betrayed her husband's tribe to kill Sisera. Judith's after she was widowed. They were wives, until.

I was a wife, *until.*

Not one thing. No unforgiveable offense. Only I have to go. Only I begin to fantasize about my own place like a lover. I trained for wiving but I'm not made to be a wife.

The *until* is a becoming. You can't become a warrior until you separate your identity from your husband's. You can't move out of the warmth of your home, culture, religion, until something shakes you free, cracks open the earth to expose your roots. I lift my roots like skirts and go.

2009

I AM TAKING LONGER AND longer walks now. It's summertime, and I'm wearing a vintage halter dress with big flowers. I walk through the Mission District. The walk clarifies. I remember the crack of joy I felt in the slim moment between Malcolm and Gabe, my long drive into the desert. My body can't make babies; that lust was snatched from me. In its place, I want to go. I want to drive until the road runs out.

Children might have calmed that need, rooted me. They might have inflamed it. I'll never know.

I've made a decision. It's a long walk home, my arms numb with fear. Through Mission District and Cole Valley and into the Inner Sunset. I'm walking and working up my courage. The day shimmers with sunlight and I am moving through terror.

In the middle of the storm that comes, my husband says, Why do you have to be so beautiful when you break my heart?

In the end, I leave because I want to leave.

It is like withdrawal from an addiction. Only a trial separation at this point. I'm staying at a friend's place. I sit in my room and twist the ring on my finger around and around. I slip it off and on again. Off. I put it on the dresser and go out for groceries. My thumb worries the space it left behind. I feel sobs rise in my chest and have to hurry back, sit down again on the edge of the bed and cry and let myself shake. I put the ring back on. Didn't get groceries. Try again.

My window is ground level, facing the street. It's a vicious part of town. People shelter against the walls at night, fights almost every morning at three a.m., four a.m.; I wake to breaking glass and drunk voices, drunks exasperated with the hideous task of staying alive another day. I feel it all, even a dark joy that I can be this close, glass and the grate over the window the only thing separating me and them. I am a woman alone now and the street is right outside. I am skinless but alive.

In a text, I ask Gabe what he believes is his purpose in life. This is an unfair question. He answers the only way he can:

My purpose is to make you happy, he types.

In this way he has made himself a wife. To be a wife means to harness your desires, your ego, and concentrate your life's purpose in your husband.

I want something larger, I type.

I am walking home from work through the park. My body feels good, feels right. I charge up the hill, shedding responsibilities and fears as I go.

In the park is a band. It's sunset and the grass smells fat and living. I want to stay and listen, but.

But, what? I think.

Nobody is waiting for me at home. Nobody checking his watch. Nobody's disappointed or scared or miserable or angry if I get home late, if I stay in the park to listen to a band.

I listen until they stop playing, then continue my climb to the top corner of the park. I look out over the lights of the city and I am bursting with all the possibilities in front of me. I don't know yet the terrible requirements of freedom.

~

I know now I can't go back. I have to murder my marriage, drive Yael's spike clean through it.

I meet Gabe just before couples' therapy and tell him it's over. He storms in for our appointment and throws his wedding ring across the room.

Our therapist cries. She's new at this. We are all three crying at each other in her office. We are her first divorce.

Afterward, I walk into the evening. I stop at a bar and tell the bartender I just left my husband. I buy him a drink and we toast each other.

It isn't a virtue. A reflex, rumbling under my consciousness. I bend and twist myself into what I believe a man wants of me. My contortions aren't always successful or even attractive. I want to curl inside the man I love, fit precisely his wifely fantasies. When I fail I feel it like a knife between my eyes, cold and blunt. I have failed my husband. Mutilated myself to fit him, like Cinderella's sisters, and failed anyway, like them. *No* does not come naturally to me, but I am trying hard to claim it. The effort to distinguish his needs from mine is too heavy to carry. Easier to let it all crash to the ground.

I leave a long smear of blood in my wake: his and mine.

We are civilized. Like I did with Malcolm, I take little with me. There are no arguments over who gets what. I suggest how to untangle our finances and he agrees.

And then I'm gone. I can feel his grief as I go. I don't file for divorce, not yet. He doesn't seem strong enough. It will be years before I make it official.

The first time I call myself an ex-wife, it feels as delicious as the first time I called myself a wife. It's a lie, I'm not divorced, but it's also true. I am no wife, not anymore. I have killed the only marriage I managed to make.

Meanwhile, Dad expands. He has remarried and now he outgrows the house where Mom shrank and all of us grew. He smashes through the roof and makes a new room at the top, glass ceiling, glass all around. He grows until he can look out and up from a mattress on the floor of his glass room, space for his head to open out to the sky held trembling in its mountain cup.

I have been a wife just once, officially. But I have been wiving since I was a little girl.

I am good at wiving. I fail at wiving. Both are true.

I have been many wives.

I learn wiving all wrong. I learn skin and breath and sharp heat too early, but my best friend had to tell me to wash my hands after peeing, a boyfriend had to tell me to wash my socks, when I was thirty a colleague wrinkled up her nose at a microfiber vest I wore too often without washing. These are things a mother is supposed to teach you. Things a wife should certainly know.

I can cross-stitch and I once crocheted lumpy scarves for my brothers. I can make stew for ten and bread for half an army. My body knows the too-big smile of a good Utah wife, and I match a man's lust with my own. I made spaghetti for my brothers when I was ten, Mom instructing me from bed, but she fell asleep too soon and I guessed at the spices by smell. My education incomplete, left hanging.

I fidget the place on my finger where my wedding ring used to be. I'm not used to the nakedness of the finger. I shift my mother's ring from my right hand to the middle finger of my left hand. I fidget this ring the way I used to fidget my wedding ring.

Mom had long fingernails. Once, she displayed her hands for me, palm out. I touched the tip of my finger to the abstract sculptural ring on her right hand. I was beside her on the king-size bed.

Where did that come from? I asked.

I loved the ring. I thought I could never wear it. It requires long fingers, or the illusion of long fingers that comes with long fingernails. I break my nails or chew them off before they get anywhere as long as Mom's.

A friend of your father's made it, said Mom. An artist. He designed it for me.

I claimed the ring after she died, began to wear it on my middle finger. After the funeral, I sat on the bed next to Dad, in the empty space Mom had left. He touched a fingertip to the ring.

Where did that come from? he asked.

It was Mom's, I said. Don't you remember? Some artist friend of yours made it. Who was it?

Dad blinked his blue eyes.

I have no idea what you're talking about, he said.

Dad's memory has always been haphazard, getting more so with age. It means nothing. Probably nothing. But I like to imagine Mom's secret life. The mystery artist made her two very similar rings, one with a pearl, one with an orange stone. My sister claimed the orange stone, I took the pearl.

Mormons don't believe in hell. Outer Darkness is where the worst of the worst will go. No fires there. The only torture is utter isolation. You are cut off from God, from everyone you love. For Mormons, hell is loneliness.

As a wife I had status within the family. They had hope for me, hope that I might return to the Mormon fold, could live with them in the eternities. Now I'm moving backward, the old Amie resurgent, rolling from man to man, shame threatening to rise again. I have exiled myself. Cast out of marriage, out of family, out of home.

I meet a man. I've only been out of my marriage for two months. He is exciting to me. Where Gabe had no job, James has three. He is all energy and ingenuity, hypersocial and fearless. We draw sharp and fast to each other, and then I am home alone at night—I insist on at least two nights a week to myself, and fear slips under my skin.

I don't know what this fear is. That I am unlovable. That, without another person to see me, I disappear. I cease to matter. Alone in my apartment, I will disintegrate. And so, like with Gabe when I had left Malcolm, I capitulate to the fear. I call James, afraid to spend even one night alone.

Come over, I say.

James takes me to a sex club. We smoke a joint beforehand and my nerves crank high, paranoia an amplifier. But I put on a black dress and heels and take his arm as we walk up the hill.

Inside, I am one of only two or three women. A cloud of men gathers around us. Some of them are naked, tongues out lewdly, cartoonishly, cocks in hand.

James goes to the bathroom.

The crowd closes in around me. This is thrilling. This is terrifying. A penis brushes against my hand and I jump in my skin. Almost involuntarily, I hold up one hand, palm out.

The men immediately back off. A circle opens up around me.

It's like the kids' game Red Light/Green Light. I can say *Yes* and then *No* at any point and then *Yes* again and it will be respected, consent enforced by bouncers. Stop. Go. Stop. Green light. Red light. I have never felt so powerful.

I want to laugh out loud. I feel safe here, safe among people whose names I will never know.

(Shame is here too, shame still lives with me. Shame is not enough to stop me.)

I feel generous, bountiful as Thanksgiving dinner. I offer myself joyfully. Lit, drowning in the pleasure of sacrifice.

PART 4: NOBODY'S WIFE

Every night I strain my anxious talons out
Pinning me into the air.
I practice riding winds into the dawn
Dazzling the faces of the sun.

"LAND MINES," ILA MARIE LYTLE MYER

2010

I LIVE IN A STUDIO apartment at Sixth and Market in San Francisco. The bathrooms are shared. If I was more organized, I would know the cleaning schedule. I would plan my showers when the bathrooms are freshly cleaned. Sometimes there's blood on the tiles. One day the remains of someone's soup float in the toilet, not fully flushed. A bandage trails from the trash.

On my way out of the apartment building, I turn to the right. A woman lives here on a flattened cardboard box. Around the corner are the SROs, Single Room Occupancy hotels. There are convulsive attempts to gentrify this neighborhood, but the SROs aren't going anywhere. The SRO is one step up from the street. You get enough money for a night in one, you have a pinkie-hold.

In an SRO, you are not allowed to have a guest in your room. You are not allowed to cook. It is a bed, nothing more. So everything happens on the street. All the socializing. All the sex. All the everything. The street is full of people with no more than a square of cardboard or people half a step away from a square of cardboard or people who prey on those with no more than a square of cardboard and a bare shred of sanity.

I give a dollar to the woman who blocks my way on the street, and she kisses my cheek. It feels motherly, this kiss.

If it wasn't for us, I say to friends, my mother could have been her.

When I say *Us*, I really mean Dad. Dad would have taken care of her until the day he died.

Possibly, he also helped keep her chained to her bed.

I am not a wife with a husband to care for me, so I can't afford to sink the way she did. I see what waits: A flattened cardboard box. A blowjob in the alley below my window. A voice rising in the dark when I'm drifting to sleep: I want to die, says the voice, I want to die, I want to die.

I move into a studio apartment in the building next door with James. It's too soon, I know it's too soon, and yet I do it anyway. I've asked James to hold me lightly. He grasps. I talk about applying for graduate school somewhere far from San Francisco, and his panicked face chokes me.

We go to sex clubs and share our bodies with men, women, people outside and beyond the binary, and still, he wants a wife.

We have it all wrong. The story about women and men and who we are to each other. We think it's about men's strength and women's weakness. Maybe it was, once. A certain kind of strength that made husbands and wives. But that brand of strength is obsolete, becoming more obsolete by the moment. We are still told that the woman is incomplete without a husband, but the whole story was invented to fill the man's own lack. Eve was created so Adam wouldn't be alone. The granting of status to a married woman, the romantic storylines, polygamy, all of it—ultimately exists to save men from the terror of loneliness.

A man can't own these soft places because he's supposed to be tough. A wife fills in the ego holes, she tells him what he needs to hear, and when she doesn't or can't, a void opens beneath his feet.

I say this with all tenderness toward men. It is as dangerous to a man to admit his weakness as it is for a woman to claim her freedom.

I'm on a bus. It's dark outside and the bus is lit up inside. I'm talking with an elegant white-haired woman in a black turtleneck, silver jewelry.

I don't want a husband or a boyfriend, I tell her. I want lovers.

Be careful what you wish for, she says.

I'm not alone enough. I'm not done leaving. Not done tearing out my roots. I rid myself of apartment, job, boyfriend. I become a freelancer, and there it is, right inside the word: free.

I am sick with fear, but this time I run full-tilt into the terror. I will pick up my bed and walk, like Jesus commanded in the book of John.

I give up all my things, pack a suitcase, and begin to travel.

I lived in an apartment and had furniture and a boyfriend and a full-time job, *until*.

A new tattoo with lines from "Song," by Adrienne Rich. On my left shoulder:

If I'm lonely

Down my back:

it's with the rowboat ice-fast on the shore
in the last red light of the year
that knows what it is, that knows it's neither
ice nor mud nor winter light
but wood, with

On the inside of my right arm:

a gift for burning

I've inked this onto my body to remind myself: I am choosing solitude on purpose. I will need this reminder, will read the words again and again, whisper them to myself in the mirror. Like the rowboat, I will burn bright.

I want to fling myself as far as possible, be alone and then more alone, alone where I know nobody and don't speak the language, alone where I can't call home, have no place anymore to call home. I want to sit with loneliness until I get underneath it. There is a keen pleasure in that space: no longer sharing my breath with one person; I see all the people around me in their apartments, on the street below, in the grocery store; I see connections running from one to another, a bright web that spans the globe.

I have packed up all my things, shrunk my possessions to fit into a suitcase, and my feet have lifted me into the world.

I'm in Montevideo, and here it is. Loneliness. Solitude. One flips into the other in a flash. I'm thrilled to be alone and then I want to tear my own organs out of my body. My hands shake when I realize I don't know where I'll be in two months, don't know if I'll have work or a home. No savings, no net, I think. My heart ices over. Humans need to touch ground, need home and family and certainty. But there is no such thing as certainty, and no place is safe, not even, certainly not, home.

And then I find the next place, and breathe again.

I'm made for this. I've finally taken flight.

I am walking downstairs in traditional Uruguayan rope-soled shoes. One foot slips on the ceramic tile and I think:

I am not slipping.

Okay I've slipped, I think, but I am not falling.

I seem to fall very slowly, my thoughts have time to form like comic strip thought bubbles above my head.

I'm definitely not landing badly, I think. I am not, god help me, hitting my head.

And my head hits the edge of the step with a hollow *klok*.

I come to sprawled on the stairs. I am alone. No Gabe, no James to rush me to the hospital. I get to my feet, wobble to the door, hail a cab.

El hospital, I say.

At the hospital, I speak English and Spanish with the doctor. I've forgotten the word for *stairs*. My fingers become legs, and I walk them down imaginary stairs.

Escalera, says the doctor.

After the tests, she tells me I have a concussion.

Do you have a husband? she says.

No husband, I say.

She tells me to have friends watch me. I am to call her if I start to "throw out."

Throw up? I ask.

She nods, tells me I am to call if my friends find my speech is slurred, if I seem confused.

The next few days are dangerous, she says.

The woman I'm staying with is out of the country. I haven't made any friends yet.

My friends will take care of me, I say.

Solitude is hazardous, but I can do this. I ask the women at the cupcake shop where I write to let me know if I seem confused. They nod, serious. They know me well enough to bring my coffee as soon as I sit down, to laugh at my toddler-level Spanish, to praise me as it improves. They will know if I need help.

I took care of myself after a concussion, and I am high with my own strength. I feel free of the old story, reveling in my solitude. I spin the globe and land my finger someplace new. I step off a plane and the smell of another country is bright inside me. The first few days a terror, but then I begin to learn the language, I push out into the city alive with its strangeness. Men with guns across their chests outside a small grocery store. A shepherd, cell phone in hand, running in big steps down the hill with his flock. Narrow twisting streets in a city built centuries before cars were invented. If I spend too much money I'm the only one who suffers. I decide what to eat, where to go. I have nobody to share my embarrassment, nobody but strangers to witness my clumsiness in a new language.

From Montevideo I take a ferry to Buenos Aires and decide to stay an extra two days. That easy. Nobody is disappointed. Maybe, nobody cares. I am as unencumbered as a bullet.

~

It occurs to me that the lesson of my childhood was not how to be a wife, or not only that. It was also how to be alone.

My Uncle Stan looked like the Marlboro man. He was Mom's youngest brother and every time I saw him my heartbeat cranked high. A kid crush, sure. But my crush was romantic in the larger sense. I didn't want him. I wanted his story.

Uncle Stan in his jeans and aviator shades, mustache that hung below the corners of his mouth, a shadow of whiskers on his chin. He parked his little trailer next to our house on one visit and opened the door in back to show me inside, doll-size kitchen and bunk that looked too short for his long legs. He talked around the sinful cigarette in his mouth, telling me how to care for the baby jackrabbit I found. Our cat had killed the mother and mauled the baby now suffering in a cardboard box.

You have to give it milk from a little dropper, said Uncle Stan, squinting against his smoke. You have one of those? And keep it out of the sun, but give it a little blanket or something to keep it warm.

Uncle Stan had been married seven times, but now he was single, driving around the west in his little truck trailer. My own uncle was the goddamn cowboy in the movie, riding free and alone. If I wasn't cursed to be a little girl I could be him, and maybe I could anyway. Stan kissed me and I almost drowned in the exotic smell of cigarette smoke, his whiskers bristling against my cheek. I waved as he drove off into the literal sunset.

The jackrabbit died a few days after he left. Uncle Stan was a charming fraud and petty grifter, seven failed marriages under his silver belt buckle and then one of his former wives married him a second time. His charm nearly bulletproof but not quite. She divorced him again, realized it was safer to love him from a reasonable distance that began at her own property line.

After Grandma and Grandpa died, Uncle Stan lived alone on the ranch. His ex-wife, the one who married him twice, lived nearby. When she didn't see him for a couple of weeks she went looking for him at the ranch.

Uncle Stan, romantic hero of the lonely Western movie in my head, was dead at the edge of the property, his body already starting to rot. He was on one side of a fence, his shotgun on the other. There was an investigation but it was ruled an accident; he'd leaned the gun against the fence and as he climbed over, it fell and shot him in the head.

This, you understand, is what it is to be alone.

I'm back in Oakland for two months. Have been traveling the world a few years now, I believe I know how to carry myself. An older man at the grocery store is gentlemanly. I am fooled by this. He takes pickles down from a high shelf for me. He offers me a ride. I get into his black SUV and he takes me home. I wonder briefly if I should let him know where I live, but push the thought away. He's telling me about his wife, his grown son, his art.

Here, I say.

I—, he says. May I use your bathroom?

I can't deny a man a bathroom.

Of course, I say.

I lead him up the steps to the apartment I'm subletting. I show him to the bathroom and go on to the kitchen to put away the groceries.

He doesn't close the bathroom door.

This is odd. I choose to ignore it.

He comes out of the bathroom and puts his hat on the bookshelf. He is a giant, I think. The size of two of me. He fills the apartment. I take one step away from the kitchen and I'm in the main room. The mattress on the floor in the middle of the room.

He moves quickly for such a large man. He has both my wrists in one large hand. He sits me down on the mattress.

What follows is a comedy. My brain takes a minute to catch up. I think, *This is a misunderstanding.*

No, I say.

Don't worry, he says.

But I don't, I say.

Of course, he says.

I need to work, I say.

Yes, he says.

I am objecting and he is agreeing with me. I say no and he agrees. Meantime he is doing what he likes with me. It costs him no effort to keep my wrists pinned. His hand is enormous. No effort. He lets go long enough for me to pull away and get up, and then he pulls me back down. He is enjoying the game.

He reaches up and under my skirt. Twists my panties out of the way and his fingers are inside me.

I'm a visual person, he says. I just want to look.

But he isn't looking.

His fingers are jabbing.

I'm twelve years old again.

When I lived in Seattle, I took a self-defense class. The teacher was a former policeman from the former Soviet Union. Cops in the USSR weren't allowed to carry guns, but gang members had guns. I learned how to disarm someone with a gun. I learned how to hurt someone bigger than me. I think about the moves I learned, moves that might still be in my body. The open-handed punch to the nose, sending bone shards into the brain. Fingers in the eyes.

I could do it.

I don't.

My brain still thinks this is a misunderstanding. My body believes it's a matter of civility. And if I miss, if I don't execute it exactly right, I will have an enraged giant in my apartment.

All of this happens in my head.

Meanwhile, I struggle pointlessly against his grip.

It is strangely interesting. I am really trying to free my hands. And I can't budge. No give at all. My feet are still free, my teeth, but I don't think about them. I'm amazed that my hands are taken out of the equation so easily.

He opens his pants with his other hand. I shake my head at his crotch.

No, I say.

No, of course, he says. It's okay.

He takes my hand and puts it on his penis, through his boxers. He masturbates, using my hand. We are both on the mattress on the floor and he is masturbating with my hand.

I am not remembering my lover Andras on this mattress, just two days ago. The world of this mattress, this apartment holds two realities, and I am the fulcrum between them. A lover and naked and an excess of joy, arms above my head, the skin at my stomach thrumming with heartbeat, the well of my hips, eyes on his face, painfully bright with the force of our connection. Two days ago. Now I do not look. My dress is yanked up around my hips. I feel this stranger's penis harden in my hand, feel semen race through it. He comes in his shorts.

I close my eyes and he gets up, goes to the bathroom. Again he leaves the door open. After, I see his hand reach for his hat.

I hope I haven't transgressed, he says.

And he leaves.

Transgressed. The language of my childhood. The language of religion. I deadbolt the door behind him and lean against it, laughing. *Now* I lock the door.

I sit down and try to write about what just happened. *Bully*, I write. *I was bullied*.

My hands go still.

Enough. I get up and walk down the street to the bar. I have a drink. Another drink. Another. I start home and it's night. I don't want to go back to the apartment. There's an Ethiopian restaurant below my apartment, we share the washer and dryer. I go there. It's late, I'm the only customer. I talk to the woman behind the bar about travel, about food, about Ethiopia. Her brother joins the conversation. They tell me I must come to Ethiopia with them. They tell me I will be welcome, they tell me it will be like family. Tonight they feel like family. I am drunk. The young man, the bartender's brother, helps me up the stairs to my apartment. I lean against him. He puts his arms around me. He asks if he can kiss me.

Oh. I tell him, Not tonight. Something bad happened today, I say. A man wouldn't leave my apartment, I say.

I'm so sorry, he says. He helps me into bed. I'm crying.

Don't worry, he says.

In the moment, I don't notice the parallel.

He tucks me under the blanket on my mattress, squeezes my shoulder, and lets himself out. I spin with drink on the mattress on the floor, in lonely dark.

The next morning I open my eyes and lean my forehead on the floor.

Fucking idiot, I say. Fuck. Fuck.

I remember the young man helping me up the stairs. Only a few hours and already I'm letting another man into the apartment. I don't know what I was trying to prove, except that the first man was an exception. I was trying to prove I wasn't wrong to let a man into my apartment. It was just the wrong man.

Or maybe I wanted to prove I didn't care what happened to me.

Andras calls. It takes me by surprise. I answer and let him talk. I'm not going to tell him about yesterday. I can't tell him. I did something wrong. I'm guilty. He doesn't want to hear about this. He is a lover, not a boyfriend, I'm free to do what I want, but I feel like I cheated on him.

I tell him.

I use the word *bully*.

He says *assault*.

That was sexual assault, he says.

I am so relieved to hear these words I start to cry on the phone.

You need to get out of there, he says. Sit tight.

Within the hour he's found me a place to stay with friends in Berkeley.

I have never met these people before, but they have a studio behind their house. A studio with a bed in a garden in Berkeley. I talk to the woman about what happened. She tells me about the time when she was much younger, in a car with a man who started touching her.

When he pulled out a knife, she says, I was relieved. It made the situation very clear, she says.

This is when I know I have to go to the cops. The whole dance. A photo lineup and a statement and I'm telling them the story and I know how it sounds. I know the chances that anything will come of it are thin. I am telling the facts, all of them, even the facts that don't make me look good. They good-cop-bad-cop me. I tell them how I thought of fighting back, using the moves I'd been taught, but I didn't know if it would be enough to disable him or just make him mad.

A judge would consider it self-defense, says the younger cop.

I open my mouth and then close it. Can't begin to know how to tell him, the law does not even enter into it.

I go through all of this and I know nothing will come of it. But I want the complaint on file. This man has done this before. He will do it again. I want a paper trail.

I am fine. I tell myself I am fine. But I am like the cartoon character who is shattered and doesn't realize it right away, not until he shivers into a thousand pieces. I move on: Chicago, New Orleans, Boston, but my belief is shaken. I am too old for this. I should have known better. This is only what I deserve. A wife is protected in a way that I am not. I placed myself outside the safety of marriage. Stupid enough to allow a strange man into my apartment.

I will always be the girl on the floor under Dave H. Oh, now it all roars back. It's been there, rotting, ever since. I am the girl who thought she was going to a party, the girl aching between her legs as she walks home. Always, always, the girl on her cousin's lap. No wonder I'm alone. I'm unlovable and shameful in my bones.

I tell this story once, twice, three times. I tell it in poetry and prose. Like Yael's story, it ripples out from my center and backward and forward through my life, it fingers out into the streets around me, invades the lives of others.

Until now, I have happily shared my body however I wished. I found what I thought was the formula for health: get outside, keep moving, run, dance.

Make love. Wear what you like. A dress that feels scandalous in Montevideo magically transforms to dowdy and conservative in Buenos Aires, same dress, same me.

But I am no longer the same. I am changed. My body my enemy. My own mind a traitor. I am still working, still traveling, I pull a smile onto the front of my face but it isn't that open Utah smile, it's a muscle memory. And when I am alone, even to go to the bathroom, deep heaves pull up from inside me, I hide my face and feel it move through me like weather, then reaffix the smile, emerge.

I am trying still to be the happy slut. A lover touches me and I don't recoil. But there is a delay. I know how to motion through lovemaking, but I am not conscious I don't want it until after, until my body shudders as though the electrical impulses took this long to move from cunt to brain.

This has always been the story. *Pretty Woman* redeemed by a man who changes her life by wanting her. Marriage, then baby. Or baby, then marriage. I kick against this, picture myself actually kicking a booted foot to bring down the walls of mindless heteronormative coupling.

But in the aftermath of another breach of my body, I begin to wish for it again. Someone to protect me. Someone to make me safe. I am too alone, too exposed.

I begin to say I would stop traveling, for Someone. For a partner. A husband, or Husband Lite.

(For Andras, the lover who found me a safe place after I was assaulted. I would stop traveling, I think, for him.)

Well. I still have further to go. The raw joy of my early traveling is wounded, but all the sharper for the scar.

Yael's story in the bible is echoed in the story of Judith. Judith is a war widow. She walks into the enemy camp, passing herself off as a defector. She does her hair up, puts on her sexiest dress. She meets the general, Holofernes.

Judith knows how to flirt. Holofernes wants her. He goes to her tent and she chops his head off, drops it into a bag of meat.

So she took the head out of the bag, and shewed it, and said unto
them, behold the head of Holofernes, the chief captain of the army of
Assur . . . and the Lord hath smitten him by the hand of a woman.

Judith had to be a widow to become a warrior. She and Yael are walking beside me, these two women who rose from the ashes of their marriages to become giants.

Mom's ring is not just beautiful; it's dangerous. The silver rises to vicious points. My left hook could take an eye out.

These are my warrior years.

I begin walking alone at night, like my little girl self in Paris. No matter where in the world I am, what neighborhood, how late. Night is when loneliness expands and the walls of an apartment can't contain it. I begin to listen to the old voice that tells me I brought the latest assault on my own head. Foolish to think I can move alone in the world. At night I can sit home and drink wine and cry, I can call someone to break my solitude, or I can get outside.

People tell me it's dangerous to walk alone at night. But all these invasions of my body happened in daylight, in a place that was supposed to be safe. My cousin, Dave H, the man of the not-party, the man at the grocery store. My home, my campus, my hometown, my apartment. The sun shone and my body was breached, broken into, used. The nighttime monsters I imagined when I was a kid turn out to be ordinary men who unveil their obscene power in the day.

The silence at night calms me. I steer my feet away from late-night bars. I can hear my footsteps and there is a kind of pact with the few other night-walkers I encounter, we nod but give space, allow each other our privacy.

My mind can't stop spinning. I see bright yellow doorways, chairs on café tables, people up late behind their windows, sleeping dogs. It feels like being in on a secret. In the dark I am in communion with the breathing whole of the universe. My solitude shifts back to a sense of rightness. When

I die I will not go to a gold and marble kingdom in the sky. Instead I will merely transform into dirt, to fertilizer, to another living expression of the universe. This is a different face of the heavenly mother I once called to. She was a wife, a helpmeet to God; but in the green scent of a nighttime lawn I feel a Mother who belongs to no one. She is an intimate goddess, feral, large enough to hold me and everything I can ever imagine.

Early in the new year, I go to a sex party with a friend. She and I have been to other parties like this together. We were both experimenting, both exploring the world after marriage. We would go together for courage, though I was inhibited in her company. I preferred going alone back then, when sex with strangers felt something like love. This one is in a Victorian mansion in San Francisco. People wear masks and leather and pose on red velvet tuffets and whip each other and get whipped. People watch and people perform and people kiss in darkened corners.

And it all strikes me as ridiculous.

Worse, too aggressive, too performative, too blunt. Before, I keyed into others right away; there was communication, a gentle kind of empathy, a shared effort toward pleasure. Tonight feels like a blow. It's all wrong. I touch my friend on the shoulder and tell her I have to go. I ask her if she's okay staying alone, she asks if I'm okay walking alone. I tell her walking alone seems the best possible thing to do.

I walk home through the night, take a detour to make the walk last. It's that deep silent hour long after the bars have closed and before the early risers are off to work. Out here there's nearly enough room for me, I take in a breath and feel it roar between buildings, in and out of the spaces between my ribs.

My Utah face is split open, underneath is something ugly: I am angry with my mother. It isn't possible. This is a secret I've kept from myself. Mom should have protected me. She didn't, and I have never forgiven her. She and everything around us groomed me to give myself over, my cousin's lap simply part of my education, and his. He was young too, barely a teenager. What happened didn't have to scar so deeply. But the story piled shame on my girl shoulders, and I knew I had to keep it secret. I knew it meant my ruin, not his. By the time my mother finally asked, I wasn't surprised that her concern was for him, for the state of his soul. We were both taught to protect our virtue but not our hearts; not our joy; never, never our freedom. All these years, I'd turned my white-hot anger against myself for failing to stop what happened.

It's telling that I am not angry with my father.

Protection, my subconscious brain says, is a mother's job. A woman's job.

But look at this: "Anger," says Adam Phillips (*Unforbidden Pleasures*), "is hope: hope that things can be different; that frustration can be modified."

Maybe not hope, exactly. But you can't be angry unless you believe things *should* be different. My whole life I've believed the world around me was as it should be: I was the one who was wrong, misaligned. I am angry now. Finally, I believe in a different possibility. I have to keep going.

Istanbul is larger than I can quite hold in my head. I take the tram, a bus, a ferry, the subway, another bus, and still I'm in the city. My neighborhood is conservative, majority Muslim. I feel exposed with my hair uncovered, and the only bars are Man Bars. I'm out for a nightwalk, stop outside a man bar to take a picture through the glass door. In the time it takes to pull phone from purse, two men have closed in fast. One comes outside, stands close to me. The other fills the door on the other side of the glass.

Buyurun, says the man beside me. He might be telling me to fuck off.

I show him my phone. I make my eyes big and Utah-innocent, try to tell him in infant Turkish that I only wanted to take a picture.

He steps back, lets me snap a photo.

My heart is beating madly as I walk away.

But I took the photo. I am walking alone at night in Istanbul. I am still alive. I'm badly broken, the shards of my brain in confusion, but I am still alive.

I'm on a crowded tram. It's night. I'm facing the dark windows, standing. I feel something thrust against my ass. In the window reflection I can see perfectly. Behind me to the left is a woman with an enormous purse. To the right a man in a sleeveless leather vest, heavily tattooed, weightily muscled. One of his hands holds the strap above my head, the other invisible. It might be the woman's purse. It might be the man. Eighty-five percent of me wants to ignore it. It's the purse. Let it go. Don't call attention to myself. But the something new in me won't let this pass. I widen my stance, force some room around myself in the crowd, throw my right elbow back, as though by accident, directly into the midsection of the big man. His eyes jump to mine, reflected in the window. I do not look away. My freshly discovered anger rages up and out. I put all of it in my face, in the look I fire into the reflection.

Do not mistake, I think at him. I am not fucking around.

Anger is hope.

The man's lowered hand immediately jumps to join his left hand on the strap. He scoots and arcs his body to put as much space as humanly possible between us, though there is little give in the crowd. At the next stop, he disappears. I think he's gotten off the tram. A few stops later, the crowd thins enough for me to see to the far end of the car. He's there, cowering in the corner.

This is not an exaggeration. This man in all his leather and muscle is cowering. I pin him again with my naked Utahless face, and he gets off the tram.

At her feet he bowed, he fell, he lay down.

As an unmarried woman, I've regressed to a kind of pre-adulthood. In Sri Lanka, women in their twenties will call me Sister, while a woman my own age is Auntie.

You're Sister, Mana will say, because you aren't married.

I know I am an adult. I support myself, make my way alone in the world. But I live in other people's spaces. I house sit, pet sit, rent a room. I move through other marriages as a quasi-child of the family, a stranger, an interloper. Having no home of my own renders me visibly dependent, even when I am paying rent. I must monitor my behavior, my neatness, my personal odors to please the rightful owners of the space I occupy. A bad review on Airbnb can drown my chances of finding a home in the next port.

I am as anxious to make myself the perfect guest as I once tried to make myself an ideal wife.

I stay two, three months in any one place. About the length of a tourist visa, but I avoid tourists. I stumble my way through unfamiliar languages, my tongue like rocks in my mouth. In every place, I try to imagine myself settling into a tidy little house here, or an apartment with bright windows. I imagine getting married again, dreaming in this language, growing old, dying here.

2015

I'M IN LOVE. ANDRAS, THE man who found me a place to stay after the assault. I've been traveling and making love with whoever I want, straight or queer, but I have held this love inside me everywhere I went. It's a gradual realization: he's more than a lover. It's a difficult love and maybe this appeals to me. I feel we are approaching each other closer, or I am approaching him. I approach him carefully, as one approaches a wild animal.

Not carefully enough. One night he tells me he has to step back. He loves me, but he cannot be a partner. He loves me, but.

Maybe this time I was the one who was grasping. The wifeness doesn't go so easily.

The next morning, realization sinks into my body as I wake. If I do not move, what happened last night will not be true, I can hold onto the pretty fantasy of togetherness I'd built in my head. I stay as I am, pinned into bed. Daylight leaks into the room around the blind, but if I close my eyes, if I pull myself deeper under the sheet, it won't get on me. I'm past crying. My body is heavy, each joint a locus of gravity. I could stay here in bed forever, like Mom in her darkened room. The story I had been fighting back rushes in on me, true all along. I am not worthy of love. This person I love so much made a choice, and it wasn't me.

I thought heartbreak would be easier to bear as a grown-up.. I have never, in all my heartbreaks, felt so broken. Maybe everything gets heavier as you get older. Maybe I'm not a grown-up after all.

The only thing that gets me out of bed is the thought of razor blades. I will find a pharmacy, I think. I will buy razor blades.

Virginia Woolf writes, "The creature within . . . cannot separate off from the body like the sheath of a knife or the pod of a pea for a single instant."

My body: this phrase a fundamental lie. A double lie, the possessive *my*, the othering of *body*. Like Woolf, I see it, a keen revelation: I am the same point in space and time as my body, my consciousness is my skin, eyelashes, belly, knees; this whole walking jumble of physical thingness is me, and more. No hard line between skin and air, this sack of skin another lie, an illusion; I have no edge but in every instant I am exchanging molecules with the air around me, sheet, street, socks and shoes, exhaust from a passing car, other human creatures in their non-finite sacks of skin. The *I* encompasses all of this and as I walk I feel eyes open, *I*'s open all up and down the street, apertures to a divine breath; I am part of this moving shifting glittering whole and the words that held me down in that bed, *sin, unworthy, unloved, selfish, slut*, spin out into gibberish.

Woolf understood this, and still she ended herself.

I am not Virginia Woolf. I am not my mother.

I want coffee.

I sit down in a coffee shop and order coffee, nothing has ever tasted so live, the coffee round and plumped out with real cream. I am stripped of all hopes, all fantasies; I may still buy razor blades, but first this, there is nothing bigger in this boiling world than a single, perfect cup of coffee.

Quietly, almost without notice, I go on living.

My sister tells me what Mom was like when Leda was little, when Mom was healthier. The Mom I only knew from home movies, in pedal pushers and sunglasses presiding over a birthday party in our backyard. That Mom was harder, glossier. Back then Dad would bring her dinner from Sizzler while the rest of us ate macaroni and cheese.

She still had special food set aside for her in the fridge when I was growing up. We all stole sips from her cans of Fresca.

Mom and Leda clashed hard by the time Leda was an adolescent. My perfect sister. I had no idea what they could fight about. One night I was playing under the dinner table after one of their awful fights, and two ladies from the church came over. Mom leaned in and told them that Leda had made her pass out. She looked so delighted to be the victim in this story.

Our brothers experienced a different, warmer Mom. Like me, she had been trained to focus her love on men; women were competition. Even her own daughter. But she had softened by the time I came around.

It's terrible to think that Mom had to get sicker before she could show maternal love toward a daughter. Even so, I moved in the shadow of her romance with Dad. I never felt like I got enough attention.

Maybe nobody ever does.

I drag myself from bed to self-defense class. Krav Maga, a particularly ugly, efficient form of street-fighting. Do maximum damage, get out fast. Class takes my body to panting, heaving exhaustion. I'm too old, too out of shape, feet bad with plantar fasciitis. Half the size of my sparring partners, I can't afford it, and I love it. There is an aptitude, hidden inside the folds of Utah Nice, a person who fights dirty, unbeautifully, unfairly. The girl who bit and scratched her brother. The girl who lost her temper with the neighbor boy, two years older than her, and pushed his dickish blond head into his shoulders, pushed with all her girl-monster force until his face turned stoplight red and tears shot out. An especial facility for dealing with multiple assailants, the strategy of using one as a shield from another comes easily—four brothers to one sister, geometry built in early. When the instructor has me lie on the floor while four other students— all young men—pile on top of me, my brain warms with familiarity. Nostalgia.

Dog pile on Amie!

I fight my way to my feet in twenty-five seconds.

Do not imagine that I picture anyone's face on the heavy bag. The instructor says I must be working something out when he sees the force of my punches, the bleeding knuckles, but it isn't so straightforward. Or maybe it's simpler: salvation lies, again, in the body. It's a start.

I need to put space between myself and Andras. I need to free myself of my neediness. I have not reconciled my opposing selves: I want to be alone, but still I want the validation I associate with being a wife, being chosen. I still hang an expectation of emotional safety on a marriage, or quasi-marriage, but I don't know if I could ever live with someone again.

I imagine the farthest corner of the world. I imagine a place that almost seems like a fairy tale. I imagine sharp, clear air in the tops of Nepali mountains.

A long plane ride to China, change planes in Guangzhou, from there to Kathmandu. I'm crying as my flight rises above San Francisco at night, tears running sideways toward my ears as though I'm heading into the wind.

We fly through a day and a night and into day. I step out of the plane into a place so different my head feels trepanned, brains exposed in the cup of skull, eyes straining from their sockets, every part of me extended to take it all in. This is not keen mountain air. Kathmandu is a big city, but almost none of the streets are paved. Each Tata truck, scooter, and car plumes its own dust creature; murmurations of dust billow into sky from wheels. And in the gaps, a city that looks halfway between disaster and rebuilding, exposed rebar on the roof of every house as though the whole city expects to add another floor any day now, elaborate piles of bricks, blue and mandarin orange and purple: walls, sarees, kurtas.

I am changing for bed when I hear a harsh whisper over my left shoulder. Shush, it says. I freeze where I am. There is nobody here. No. It was nothing. The sound of pajamas shushing over socks.

I know that is not how that sounds.

Someone is in my room. Someone is in my room or I am hallucinating. Both possibilities sicken me.

I look over my shoulder and the floor of the room tilts upward, shakes itself like a dog trying to dislodge me from its back, and the blood horror that rises in me is real as a just-sharpened blade. I crouch, then go facedown on the floor, holding on with both hands.

Down here with me is a fly.

The fly walks easily along the tilting surface, up and over my hand.

This fly is a gorgeous creature. Long-bodied. Narrow wings. I bring my face closer. Striations along the length of the wings, a delicate veining. Fly wing, leaf, hand. The noise in my head stops, shut off like a choir when the director closes his hand. Fly and me. Floor just floor. I am lying on my belly. My nose almost touching those faerie wings, I will not let my breath disturb this insect savior, winged angel, meditation. Fly wings, fly eyes, busy fly legs.

You and me, Fly. Show me the way.

I am assigning a gender to the fly. She is a she. I keep my eyes on her. I am interested in this fly, like a toddler distracted from a tantrum. I look at her and my breath calms.

I'm on a train, Sri Lanka. A train from Colombo aiming deep into the countryside. It was sunset when we left Colombo. It's nighttime now. The train has emptied. I'm not sure how close we are to Puttalam. I get up to rummage through my bag, and I see:

I am not alone.

A man in a red shirt stands at the back of the car, in the corridor between cars. He is looking at me and jacking off.

I sit down quickly. My body gets ready to fight. It is forever. A train disappearing into the Sri Lankan countryside, deep, yellow-mooned night, man in a red shirt.

I hear something, a half-breath, and I look up. The man is standing in the aisle beside my seat. He opens his mouth to speak.

I hold up one finger like a schoolteacher, and shake it at him.

This is a small thing.

One finger.

He hangs his head like a chastened schoolboy, slinks back to a seat several rows back.

As we approach a stop and I duck to read the sign, he pipes up from his seat: Not Puttalam, he says.

He is helping me. He heard me earlier tell a young couple I was going to Puttalam. He is going to help me.

We ride longer into this endless night, he in his row, me in mine. At each stop he says, Not Puttalam, until at last at last: Puttalam.

I want to be relieved that a young man has been sent to meet me at the station. He gives the name of the place where I will be teaching English as though it is a password, and so I climb into his tuk-tuk.

The best tuk in all Sri Lanka! he says. Look in back.

I turn to see enormous speakers behind my seat.

We will rock! he yells over the ruckus of wind as we pick up speed.

For once, I did the right thing by shaking my finger at the man in the red shirt, and he was, astonishingly, shamed by my performance of virtue. I am proud of myself. And I blame myself, again, for somehow inviting this.

A different man, a different situation, and my act would have meant nothing.

Now I am hurtling down the road in a cloud of stadium rock with another man I do not know, and he brings me safely to the quiet village.

While I am here in Sri Lanka, Andras messages me. Carefully, tenderly, we begin to rebuild a friendship.

I fly back to California, touching ground in my former home, and see Andras again. We are friends, and I am trying mightily to close off my wish for more. And then he kisses me. He begins to say he wants—not marriage—but Something, with me. I leave again: Serbia, Barcelona, a seaside village in France, and I believe he has changed his mind, that we will be different.

I begin to construct a fantasy where he will ask me to marry him, no matter that he has always called marriage a cage, no matter that he swore he would never be a husband (again). My brain hears the things he says and shapes them into occult clues; he longs to be my mate. We will have a sweet life. I nurse this idea for months, from country to country. If I bend myself just right, I think, he will realize I am made to be his wife. I will be Chosen, like the game I played with my sister, Moses in the rushes.

But in our long phone conversations, I feel him pulling back again. My fantasy chokes, the happy couple illusion disintegrates for good. When I return to the US, I am crumbling, too.

I've been invited to an artists' residency in Arizona. Bed seems the only safe place, but I know just how dangerous it is. I pull myself out of the room to get dinner. Two women who live in my dorm call to me from the shade of a tree.

Our dorm is haunted, says one.

It's La Llorona, says the other.

La Llorona, the ghost who sobs eternally for the children she murdered.

I heard sobbing coming from Room 6, says the first.

Nobody lives in Room 6, says the second.

Oh, I say. *I* live in Room 6.

They look at me.

I'm La Llorona, I say. I laugh.

La Llorona is too apt. My body murdered my never-were children before they could exist. I haven't had a period in twelve years, ever since my uterus was taken; still my ovaries keep cranking: *make life, make life, make life.*

But my body is death. Death bloomed from me in a river of blood until the hysterectomy dammed it up. And then my mother died. And then I murdered my marriage. No romance since has survived in my harsh environment.

One night, in Room 6, I dream I'm nursing the lifeless carapace of a baby, light as rice paper.

In Arizona, finally, I file for divorce. It has been nearly eight years. I do it in hopes of stirring myself back to life.

~

I can't stay in bed, not like Mom did. There is no bed that is truly mine. There's no one in my life like my father, ready to bring me food. I get up and get outside or I starve. I get up and work or I starve. That simple.

There is, of course, a lower rung of depression, the one where starvation doesn't matter so much. I have not yet descended to that rung. It's possible that getting out of bed, getting outside, helps keep me from that lowest rung.

It's likely I just haven't found the bottom of the chemical candy bowl, not yet.

I'm depressed but it's a simple depression. Not clinical, I tell myself. Not capital-D Depression. I'm not Mom. This is what I tell myself. My heart is aching over Andras, that's all. Over the family life I can't seem to make. Anyone would be depressed.

My dizzy spells are back, Ménière's flaring up under stress. I fall down crossing the street, walking up stairs. The doctor recommends a cane. I use my cane with style, make it a part of me. But I can't avoid it: my body is breaking down again. Like Mom's. I wasn't able to keep myself forever supple with my frenetic pace.

I am dizzy, and menopausal. The doctor tells me my ovaries have finally shut down. Hot flashes in climate-change-hot July.

Next, I think, I'll go someplace cold.

Winter in Iceland, then. There are three hours of daylight every day. The sun doesn't clear the horizon at all for at least a week. It stays just behind the slope of the volcano, skims across the edge of earth, then dips into darkness. Three hours of sunset, the sky close and painted in celestial colors.

I sleep more than usual, but it's understandable. The dark tells my body it's time to sleep.

It's not depression anymore, or not as much. My heart opens out into sky as I tromp through knee-deep snow. On Christmas Day, like every day, I take a walk. I don't know anyone here, and I assume Icelanders spend Christmas inside with their families. I have no family to spend Christmas with. Since Mom died, Utah no longer feels like home. My former bedroom has been converted into an office; the downstairs remodeled to an apartment, rented out. On the rare occasions when the family gathers, we do not fill the house with our noise, do not share breakfast in pajamas; there isn't space for us anymore. I will not feel sorry for myself. Today I wander, get as lost as possible on a mile-wide island. I find myself in the cemetery.

This is what Icelanders do on Christmas, it appears. Downtown was ghosted, but there are families here and there in the cemetery. The crosses are adorned with lights. When the snow melts, I'll see extension cords snaking around the headstones. But for now the beauty is almost unbearable, these glowing bulbs in the twilight. My spirit feels too big for my body.

I cry about twice a day. If it was depression, I wouldn't be able to get myself out of bed when the wind kicks in my front door, walks heavily through the house. If it was depression, I wouldn't want to go out into the gale, where my hat whips off my head, my cane lifts, and I rise with the wind, feel myself become a giantess—a goddess—grown to match the Icelandic sagas.

I walk the long way around the island on January 20, 2017, the day of the Women's March. A one-woman march. About ready to turn back when, in the distance, I see a figure on the shore.

It's not that I want company. I'm pulled. Someone else got out there, no apparent path. Big waves crashing on the rocks. I want to be there too. Steer my feet toward the water.

As I get closer I realize the figure hasn't moved.

Not a person after all. A bronze statue of an angelic woman, floating above the surf. I step around to the front to read the inscription: *In memory of Icelanders who heard the call to build Zion and emigrated to Utah, 1854–1914.*

Mormons! I laugh out loud into the waves. Exactly here, this wild and lonely shore at the edge of a volcanic island in the North Atlantic. This statue—a celestial woman alone—is unusual for my people. I don't believe in signs. Rather a riotous joke from a god I don't believe in.

This is the longest I have ever been without a boyfriend, a lover, a husband. Why is it so hard to shake the idea that marriage equals morality? Everyone smiles at the dear old couple holding hands as they shuffle down the street. You can't help it. Love that long: a virtue. A prodigy of grace. But love is selfish, too. Guaranteed companionship. An apparent wall against loneliness.

I chose to be alone. I have friends all around the world, but I can't stop measuring my own worth according to my wifeliness.

When are you getting married? My mother's deadly half-joke.

I have a project. I'm plotting to overthrow the current US government. The presumptive president, the sexual assaulter-in-chief, our collective narcissistic bully. He treats his wives as accessories, women as toys for his pleasure, targets for his contempt. He spits *rapist* and *Mexican* in the same breath, a performance, claiming to defend white women from dark hordes swarming over our borders. The whole country is rushing backward at alarming speed, people of color and immigrants and women losing their personhood, becoming things. Again. It was always there and now it's rising back to the surface. I rage back at echoes of the religion that raised me. I rage at the people who carried him to power.

His florid face repels me. It snags my attention like a tarantula in my bed.

He sweats and brags of salacious desire for his own daughter.

His lips push out.

I feel his fingers inside me, stabbing.

I'm ready to return to the US from Iceland and save it from itself. I don't know exactly what I'll do, but I feel marvelously suited to do Something. I have nobody depending on me. Few ties. No home. I'm used to traveling and strange accommodations. I'm made for this. My larger purpose here in front of me. I imagine myself a resistance fighter. I don't know where the core of this resistance is, but I'm sure I can track it down.

I am ready to use a knife the way I threw an elbow into the man in Istanbul. Use my remaining wifely charms to seduce them—whoever they are—Mata Hari–style. I'm forty-eight but surely (surely!) I can seduce someone.

This plan seems entirely reasonable.

Maybe it isn't. I don't know how to tell.

We have made a bright line between wife, whore, victim, and set each against the other, but they all grow from the same, sticky narrative. We've tweaked the story, overlaid the idea of wife as equal partner, marriage as intimate and loving. We are reclaiming whore, women as free agents, no longer condemned for choosing to make love.

But the victim is still feared, the victim shames and terrifies us all, she lays the story wide open, the story none of us wants to acknowledge: woman was made for the pleasure of man.

Eve is still with us, all our stories built on her shoulders.

I believe I'm making a new choice. I will not be compliant, I will not exist for a man, will not be his whore or his victim. But even the assassin, even the lone woman living the cowboy myth, even she is trapped inside the borders of the story. One of my sparring partners in Krav Maga lit up with lust—he thought my violence belonged to him, too. And if it doesn't, if I dare belong to no one, we know what happens next. I walk down the street alone and men's eyes stick to me. Their eyes full of want and resentment, both at once. I will not escape punishment.

And, so? That's no reason to stop.

Back in San Francisco, and something feels different. I am angry. No, afraid. No, inconsolable. A list of grievances against Andras grows in my head. I take long walks and stage arguments with him. I'm talking to myself like an asshole with a Bluetooth headset, but I have no Bluetooth. I put my fingers to my lips, unsure if I'm speaking out loud. And then I forget how I must look, plunge back into obsessive righteousness. He doesn't care about me. If he cared, he would want to marry me, even though I don't want to be married, not exactly. My spinning brain has reverted to primitive forms: marriage would be proof of his love. He tells me he's my friend, but he trivializes my suffering. He thinks I should be over my heartbreak, that I shouldn't be heartbroken at all. He believes I am weak for wanting a partner.

I look for safety where there is no such thing, safety in a structure I don't quite believe I can support. Maybe, oh maybe, I can be a wife a second time around if he'll just give me a chance. I win every imaginary argument, I stun him into silence.

When I actually talk to him, I split him into two people: the lover who broke my heart, and the friend who tries to help me cope. The anger masses inside my chest and I lose track of what I meant to say.

Let's call him John, I say to Andras on the phone. I love this man named John, but he doesn't want me. You are my friend, Andras. Tell me what to do. John is hurting me, I say. He is pretending to care so that ... so ... I don't know why.

For a while, you did want to be my partner, didn't you? I ask. I didn't imagine it?

The truth is, I say, my words growing thick in my throat, I don't deserve to be loved.

He is talking, throwing words at me, but I won't remember most of what he says, just a rain of sound, a sense that he is characterizing me in a way that feels entirely false.

And then:

That voice in your head is a liar, says Andras. You don't have to listen to it.

He is gently trying to suggest that maybe, maybe, my mind is skittering away on its own trip.

This is real, I say. My feelings are valid. Just because I'm a woman doesn't mean I'm hysterical, I say.

I can't stop hearing Malcolm. That isn't mildew you smell. You're imagining it.

A cold fear seeps up my spine. Either Andras is right and I'm crazy, or the person I love is a misogynist asshole, gaslighting me. This is not an argument that is possible to win. I don't consider a third possibility: It is true that I have been wounded. It is also true that I am keeping the wound open; I feel driven to hurt myself over and over.

(Or, more simply, these are menopausal mood swings. I'll see a doctor and get hormone treatment. Easy do, as my father says.)

~

My divorce has been finalized without my knowing. The agency that helped with the paperwork contacts me for the remainder of what I owe, and this is how I learn it's done. I go to the courthouse and pick up my papers.

No relief, not like I expected. Far too late, too many years, too much life slipped out from under my feet. I stop at a bar for a glass of champagne, a celebration, but it's an empty performance. Dark moods still roil inside my head. There is nobody to put his fingers on my pulse, nobody to hold me while I shake. I don't miss my marriage, but loneliness grows teeth in a crisis. I am a divorced woman, menopausal, dried up. Outside, it's a quiet afternoon all through the city. I walk home for miles, from downtown San Francisco to a friend's place by the beach. I cut through Golden Gate Park and put my hand on a tree trunk, imagine I can feel life moving through it. I feel tenderness toward Gabe, but there is no doubt: my world has become bigger since I left.

A xeroxed piece of paper, folded and stashed in my bag, and it's done.

In Mormonism, it's possible to divorce a spouse who has died. As difficult as any other temple divorce. A way to spare yourself their company in the afterlife.

I am in the middle of my second life, my after-marriage life, the closest I can imagine to an afterlife, but a spouse never entirely leaves you. I carry Gabe with me, and Malcolm. And Mom, my first practice run at wiving.

I see a doctor and she says, I don't like to prescribe hormones anymore.

Prozac, she says. It's not good if you're bipolar, but it's the preferred treatment for menopause.

I tell her my mother was bipolar.

Well, you can always go off it, she says.

A suspicion crawls into my brain. Maybe this is more than menopause. (I take the Prozac.)

Many of the people I love and admire most are bipolar. It feels presumptuous to assume I have it. As though I would claim their charisma for myself.

I swing wildly between seeing bipolar disorder as horrifying (Malcolm's mom with bra and panties on over her clothing; my mother with her face creased into a static *I'm disappointed* grimace) and glamorous (Mom at her most charming; a friend's brilliant leaps from one idea to another). My mind can't admit any nuance beyond these gross characterizations. It must be one or the other.

It's Saturday night in San Francisco. I step across Twenty-Fourth Street to meet friends at the corner bar. Inside, a young couple's tangled legs show under the curtain of a photobooth, the hem of her skirt sparking in the flash. They are young enough to be my own kids, if I'd ever had any.

I can get up now and walk in front of a car, I think.

No, not car.

Train is better.

I picture an SF Muni train speeding toward me, its nose fitting smooth into the curve between hip and ribs. In hospital emergency rooms in San Francisco, there is a special code for Pedestrian vs. Muni. Pedestrians always lose.

Not Muni, I think. BART.

BART trains scream fast underground. I remember being stuck on a train while a body was cleared from the tracks. I am sitting quietly on my barstool but my body is alive with the shriek of an oncoming train.

Are you OK? asks my friend Dawn.

I smile sweetly at her.

No, I say.

I've been on Prozac for two and a half weeks, but this is new. I finish my drink and go. I don't step in front of a train, but the image won't leave my mind.

When I wake the next morning my whole body feels like it has been yanked inside out, organs splayed, blood swamping the sheets. My brain can't process the sunlight coming in the window; it's still throwing up this picture of a train. I am close to the beach, there are no BART trains out here, but I picture the train running parallel with the shore.

I go back to sleep.

My housemate Mischa calls upstairs. It's been six years since I started traveling. Mischa has provided me shelter, and I must put on a face for his sake. Dawn is making brunch for us at her place. I can't disappoint either of them. Dawn will be wearing her favorite, hilarious throwback of an apron and making something delicious. She parodies an old-fashioned wife. It takes everything I have to pull on my clothes.

A BART train screams through my head.

I sit on Dawn's couch while drinks are being mixed. I need help. I need to go to the ER, but I must be careful how I present myself. I don't want to be committed. At this particular point in time, the only thought more unbearable than the train in my head is being confined to a mental facility. I remember the comforting elsewhere of the hospital when I was sixteen. But the ability to go outside is part of what has kept me alive this long. And, not incidentally, I can't afford more than a day away from my freelance work. As long as I have to go on living, I have to work.

I stand up and tell Dawn and Mischa I'm taking the bus to the ER.

Don't be silly, they say, after their shock, after their questions. We'll take you.

What I am experiencing is called intrusive thoughts. I know the term, and I use it at the ER. Intrusive thoughts and suicidal ideation are potential side effects of Prozac. I have been narcotized, swaddled in muslin, sleeping far too much. It was decidedly unpleasant.

And then the train thoughts.

In the ER, I have to surrender all my things. I give my purse to Dawn.

She and Mischa go out for brunch and get good and drunk. Later, when I'm released, Mischa will take an Uber to pick me up.

A husband like my father, like Gabe, would have stayed in the waiting room, no matter how many hours. I hate that I think this. If Andras was waiting for me all this time, I would be nervous for him, worried about him. Maybe friends are better.

I'm set up on a chair in a hallway. I am in elephantine scrubs like the other patients here. I had to put everything into a plastic bag that was sealed and taken away, my cell phone, my notebook, my bra, my socks. One man lurks in the doorway of his room, shuffles out, holding up his scrubs like a debutante lifting her skirt, shuffles back. Two tranquilized men in two rooms snore grandly in stereo.

I have no phone, no book to read, nothing to do with my hands. I start writing in the corner of a handout I've been given. A nurse scrounges up some blank paper, hands it to me with a clipboard. Doctors come and go, talk to me, write on their own clipboards. I write, doodle, write more.

After the doctors disappear, the nurse meets my eyes.

You seem very clear about what's happening, he says. It's rare that someone comes in here with such clarity. Promise me you won't make an attempt on your life, okay?

This sounds like goodbye, but it's many hours still before I'm released. I'm next to the security guard at his station, and I overhear his conversation with an orderly.

So he leans into me, the security guard says, and he's . . . *sniiiiiiiiiifff*. And I say, Are you *smelling* me, Man?

And he says, You don't stink!

Fuckin' right I don't stink, I say.

I thought all black guys smelled, he says.

Why the hell you think that? I say.

Well, he says, James stinks.

And I'm like, James? Fuck, man. That dude doesn't know *what* a shower is. You think all black guys are like him?

And then I realize: James and me are the only black people he *knows*!

They hoot with laughter. I join in. They ignore the crazy lady in blue scrubs; I don't blame them. They are the best people in the whole world.

The ER told me to go off the Prozac and gave me exactly five Ativan. I use them as sparingly as I can, but now I'm down to just one.

My therapist suggests I time my mood swings. I can feel one as it ratchets up, like an ancient rollercoaster cranking to the top of its run. It slows at the top. I know what's coming next. No brakes no tracks no safety anywhere, I'm plunging. Adrenaline dumps into my brain and the meat behind my ribs knots tight. I want to run away but there's nowhere to run. I want to shout at someone. Anyone. I want to take their fucking head off. I want to use my teeth, feel bone and gristle in my mouth. Maybe our vicious POTUS. Maybe Andras, my dead mother, my ex-husband Gabe. Doesn't matter. The rage has to land somewhere.

I often cry. Not tender tears. Something craven, terrified, spilling over. As I walk down the street, sit in a restaurant over lunch, in front of my laptop. Anywhere.

And then it's gone. I mean gone, no aftertaste, nothing. I'm back to baseline depressed. I check my watch. Three minutes.

Two minutes of relative relief, and then I feel the rollercoaster cranking up again.

Every five minutes, all day.

I feel I'm half a step away from a square of cardboard on the street.

No, I tell myself. *It's only menopause.*

All at once I want to stop traveling. Six years is enough. My moods are yanking me viciously around and I want solid ground. In the middle of it all, I begin to make plans. I will find a place to settle, but this time it's different. I do not want to stop traveling because of a man. I can make a home without being a wife. I will go somewhere I know nobody. Start again.

The thought is as scary as traveling was when I first began.

The last time I was in Utah, Dad showed me an album he'd made of Mom. Mom in her borrowed wedding dress, cat-eye glasses. Mom running on the beach. Mom in a swimming pool, short hair wet, smile warm but uncertain. One eye in shadow. Mom, early in their marriage, when they went to France. She's lying across the hotel bed, hair bouffanted high and soft. Man's white shirt, narrow skirt. She is gorgeous. Her smile just edging toward ironic.

I'd never seen this picture before, and it hurt. She's looking directly into the camera, into me. Into Dad's eyes I guess, but I am standing now in his place and my gaze changes her—like observing a quantum particle affects its trajectory, Mom becomes a creature of my own making. Mom before her own path sloughed away all her choices, before she was shunted down the chute toward death. Now she's gone and she is my creation. More, the longer I look.

On the facing page was a handwritten note.

> *Dear Peter—*
> *I love you so much. But I am so tired, so ill, so depressed. I have lived*
> *for more than too long—Please make it possible for me to go—*
> *I don't know—can't you tell me how I can get away? Just slip away*
> *in my sleep—*
> *I'm so sorry. Please help me*

What is this? I asked.

The handwriting was crowded and spindly, lines sloping upward until the last three words. *Please help me* drags steeply toward the bottom-right corner of the page, no punctuation at its end.

Your mother wrote that maybe two months before she died, said Dad.

Dad saved this note and put it in Mom's album. I understand his impulse to save the note, to display it. It is stitched into us from birth: repentance requires confession, restitution. These heavy words. Dad has hung Mom's suffering around his own neck. He believes that he can expiate his sin by chaining himself to her accusation. That is what this letter was, a pointed finger. Mom would never have admitted to blaming him for what happened to her life, but Dad blames himself. I blame him, too. And her. And myself. All of us.

But there was a point where it became as inevitable as a death in a novel. Mom had obliterated herself, pill by pill.

~

So okay, yes, I'm cracking up.

It costs me greatly to admit this. After years with Malcolm, fighting him to hold onto my reality, fighting anyone who tried to tell me I didn't have a right to my own space, my feelings, my anything.

Now, but. I have to accept that my reality doesn't match the world outside my head.

In the meantime I get up and work every day, though I can't vouch for the quality of my work. In the meantime I get to appointments on time, or nearly on time. In the meantime I dress myself and go for walks. Five, six-hour walks. If I keep moving, I can almost keep pace with the fear.

Meanwhile my body is still grieving its loss of fertility, twelve years after my uterus was cut out of me, my interest in sex at zero. I won't so easily escape from myself in a man's bed, not anymore.

I am in a psychiatrist's office. I am paying, out of pocket, an amount I cannot afford.

I'm holding, white-knuckled, to the narrative I've spun: this is just menopause. I need something to bridge my body's mourning period, maybe as long as ten years, but there will be an end date, and afterward I'll have new power, the terrifying strength of the crone.

Afterward, I won't need anyone.

He asks very targeted questions about my personal history, family history, botched suicide attempt at age sixteen.

He asks if I got a diagnosis then.

My diagnosis was *Teenager*, I say. But somehow, the shape of his questions make me question myself. I'm not convincing.

Hm, he says. Most teenagers don't attempt suicide.

He asks about more recent suicidal ideation, before the Prozac. I don't tell him about the night a few years ago when I was having dinner with a friend. I had to fight the sudden urge to get up from the table and walk in front of a bus. I don't tell him about the razor blades.

I don't tell him because I forget. I don't tell him because it will mean maybe something more than menopause. I don't tell him because I'm embarrassed.

It doesn't matter that I've left these details out.

Any periods in your life when you didn't need very much sleep, he asks.

Yes, I say. I remember when I left Gabe, was living with James. I worked at his gallery space late into the night, then got up at 4:30, 5:00 a.m. to run.

And during this time, were you more impulsive than usual? More sexual?

I hesitate. I don't want to pathologize this time in my life, the real connections I made, if only briefly.

High-risk behavior? Several sexual partners?

Yes, I say finally. I don't say sometimes several at once.

Did you spend money you didn't have?

Like now, I think. I don't say that out loud, either.

Yes, I say.

And were you unusually productive, creative? he says.

It was beautiful. I loved the whole world. This was me at my most potent, the truest me. I saw connection running from my fingertips to the strap I held on the bus to my fellow riders to the street outside. I was a genius of universal love. I could not be a wife but I could wive the world.

That would be a hypomanic state, he says.

Pretty classic bipolar disorder, he says.

I nod.

What I want to say is *WHAT*. What I want to say is, Take that back. What I mean is I'm afraid to take in the next breath.

He has neatly dismantled my story in ten dry minutes.

Friends of mine have said they were relieved to get a diagnosis of bipolar. I am not. My hands are numb. I'm shocked. I shouldn't be shocked. I've been watching myself for signs all my life. But I managed to avoid knowing what exactly those signs were.

My internal narrator said I'd gotten away clean. I'm nearly fifty. Most diagnoses of bipolar disorder happen in your twenties. Like Malcolm used to say.

There are a number of women, says the psychiatrist, who have mild or moderate bipolar, high functioning. They don't know until it's uncovered in menopause.

Menopause ends. Bipolar never does.

Now that I am depressed, clinically, diagnosably bipolar, the glamor is gone. Instantaneously with the diagnosis.

I suspect everything I once knew about myself. My set point is happy? Really?

My entire sense of myself has been violated, I am hollow and fragile as the rice paper baby in my dream.

Hi Mom. Me too, Mom.

My travels, my push to the outer edges of the world, my warrior self—in the end none of this protected me from my mother's madness. Here is a glaring truth: the one thread in common between my failed marriage and pseudo marriages was me, and my gargantuan hunger to be free.

The romantic filter I applied to marriage, the romance of depression and bipolar disorder: all has fallen to ashes. A necessary death before the birth of something new.

Medication, then. Not Prozac. Something, says the psychiatrist, whom I hate, whom I love, something to even out those moods.

But I love my hypomanic states, I tell him.

Most people do, he says.

I don't know if he knows, if anyone can know. I thought this was me, so much a part of myself as to be undifferentiated from the body, the voice, the story that makes me me.

Your very self, then, nothing more than chemicals in your brain, sloshing over their boundaries.

I have—or had—a gift for ecstatic appreciation. I love like love can crack open the universe. A walk in the park and all the gods walk with me, pass me by disguised as a monarch butterfly, a grasshopper, a gray squirrel.

All these gushes of love, this ecstasy, transcendence, cosmic beauty. Chemical surges. Gone.

The dizzy spells are gone, too. The cane abandoned for now.

I am taking a pill every day. I try not to think of my mother, the fifty pills she took every day, her slow suicide. Just one pill. It promises to dampen my Olympian moments. But I live. And here it is, a minute later, and I live. Every morning I take a diamond-shaped pill and every day I do not fantasize about walking in front of a train.

Once I was a goddess, or I held a potential goddess inside me. My body never forgot the founding myths of Mormonism: to be a goddess, one must first be a wife. But I approached godhood in my solitude, in the keen joy of the road.

Now I am only human—but for today I am alive, by violent grace.

In the Renaissance, wealthy women had their portraits painted as Yael, holding a spike and mallet. Judith was more popular, signified by the sword she used—she is young, braceleted and perfumed, she bounces Holofernes's head in her bag of meat. I see Yael as plain and practical. A comfortable woman, if it wasn't for the bloody spike. As Sisera died, he cried:

"Behold pain has taken hold of me, Jael, and I die like a woman."

And Jael said to him, "Go, boast before your father in hell and tell him that you have fallen into the hands of a woman."

(PSEUDO-PHILO IN *LIBER ANTIQUITATUM BIBLICARUM*)

To die like a woman, at the hands of a woman, the ultimate humiliation. These women have been part of the story from the beginning, as much as Eve, as Sarai/Sarah, as Rachel and Leah. The story has always required a monster like Judith, like Yael, to stand in opposition to the wife. I can knee a man in the balls and it won't save me; it won't change the world any more than Judith did. I can be pliant and pleasing, I can make myself a wife again and that won't save me either. I've been fighting for years to break free of the story but the whole world lives inside the story; the only way out is to change the story itself.

Now

WHEN I WAS FOURTEEN, A boyfriend broke up with me. I'd lied about my age, said I was seventeen, but a friend exposed me. We were in the park where I used to play with Chrissie, at the base of the big tree. A family reunion noising in the pavilion down the slope. He told me it was over. Sunlight shone through his blond curls and he looked long into my face. Maybe, I thought, he will say something to gentle the blow.

You need to pluck between your eyebrows, he said.

A clear instruction. I saved up my money and got electrolysis. My single Frida brow now two, unremarkable. If I was to make myself acceptable, I had to remove any trace of friction in my appearance.

More instructions from men: wear more makeup, wear less, fix your nose, wear perfume, don't wear perfume, shave your legs, shave your pubic hair, wax your pubic hair, your asscrack, cut your hair, grow your hair, do something different with your hair, lose weight, gain weight.

A drunk Irishman once leaned across a table to squint at me.

You're the hairiest woman I've ever seen, he said.

The electrolysis wasn't enough. I did as instructed. Fixed my nose. Lost weight, shaved my legs. Took Accutane until my skin peeled off in sheets. Plucked my chin and waxed my upper lip. Joined a clinical trial for laser hair removal and zapped my lush bush to a tidy patch. A wish toward self-immolation, purified into a perfect wife.

Malcolm wanted me to get my tits done. He wanted me to get my nose redone, felt the first surgery left my nose imperfect. I thought about a breast job, I did. But my desire starts in my breasts—nipples touched in just the right way and I'm lit. I found my borderline here, would not willingly risk that glorious sensitivity.

Now I begin to age. Jawline tends toward jowls. Neck loose. Stomach will never be ballerina-flat again. It still pierces deep when a lover tells me he prefers large breasts, as though a woman's body was a menu you could order from. I don't know how not to take it personally, my body inseparable from my Self, but I no longer imagine I can transform to please. No more fantasies of an incision under my arm to plump up my breasts, make me more desirable at the expense of my own pleasure. A lover suggests I shave my now-scraggly bush, and I say:

No. Not for you. Not for anyone, not anymore.

The other night, I had dinner with my now-grown stepdaughter and a good friend. The bartender snapped a photo of the three of us, women in mid-laugh. Our laughter, arms around each other's shoulders, set off fireworks in my brain. (A relief. I can still feel.) Love spills over all boundaries: agape, philia, ludus, eros, pragma, philautia. We don't always get to choose the manifestation, but we can choose to drink, choose to pour it generously, promiscuously.

I was the one who ripped up my roots in a community as well as a marriage. I abandoned my friends, if not as completely as I had my husband. It was necessary for me, but left a wound.

As I've traveled, I've met people who have shaken me as deep as a romance. And then I left. Every time it tore my heart, but I can't deny it has also been the bright, sharp edge of emancipation.

Soon I will live in a place of my own, a modest apartment maybe, in a medium-sized town. I won't be able to run away so easily. My naked roots will find earth again, and I have no idea what will bloom.

~

I know this about myself: I need time alone to know the heart-squeezing shards of beauty hiding in every day. The shine off a parking meter. Heavy blossom scent when I pass a stand of flowers I can't name. Bare feet on a clean floor. The fairy-white of Mom's once-dark hair.

Things that have made the world sweet, have kept me alive this long, taught me to love when loving seems impossible.

The after-echo of a wave, water tick-ticking into sand. A pair of kids scaling a low wall, one reaching a hand to help the other. Garlic. A patch of heat on a lover's skin. Swinging sundress on a spring day. I am ached with joy. Even pleasure in the growing roar in my ears that comes before a Ménière's dizzy spell, that moment of exaltation like *The Idiot*'s Prince Myshkin just ahead of a seizure: "Suddenly amid the sadness, spiritual darkness and depression, his brain seemed to catch fire at brief moments. . . . His sensation of being alive and his awareness increased tenfold at those moments which flashed by like lightning."

An eight-year-old girl and five-year-old boy in Greece who knocked on the door of my doll's cottage. I was on my way down into depression, terror in being alone, uncoupled. These children arrived with their arms wide for hugs, *to keep you alive*, they said.

The night I walked in on my parents making love, Mom above Dad, reaching forward as if to take something off a shelf. She was naked, graceful as an arabesque.

In the very bottom of a lightless hole when I wanted only to end myself, exactly there, I found slow rapture in a walk on a wet gray day, the anticipation of coffee on my tongue, and I was able, again, to live.

I can see depression like a black, roiling mass underneath a glass floor at my feet. Just a thin sheet of glass between it and me.

That image, Mom on top of Dad, the love alive between them. The love extended to us children, but only so far. I learned this when I was taking lovers: a person has only so many hours, so much attention. Love is not subtractive, but attention is. Someone will always be left out. When Mom had a moment for me, I became the center of the universe. But those moments were few. My hunger for attention still roars in me; it's there with all the madness under my glass floor, ready to slip through the smallest crack.

This hunger is our tragedy. Stories are gushing out of women, stories like mine and not like mine. It is one thing to read statistics and know sexual violence is common. It's quite another to hear story after story, a wide roar from thousands, millions of women who live it every day and it's true: I look differently at men, now. Love comes harder now. I have to ask now, of every contact: was I just giving in?

My therapist provides a new dimension. PTSD, she says. Really, I think. But I haven't been to war.

Are you sure of that? she says.

The same medication I'm given for bipolar also helps smooth the body's history of shocks. Every hole punched into me was recorded, the tape now playing back the whole bloody concerto of my life.

How much women do, how completely we have stripped ourselves down for love, for approval, for attention, that searchlight that we believe will hold back the dark of loneliness.

And men, too. How terrible to believe you must cajole, push, *take* attention that isn't freely given. How terrible to suspect it never will be given freely. And so they must wind the clockwork inside their hearts, the fearsome tick-tick-tick that says a forced choice is in fact a choice.

1. I am single.
2. It is not a sin to want to be married or partnered.
3. You can have long-term intimacy without subsuming your identity.
4. It is not a sin to want to be single.
5. It is not a tragic story for a woman to be alone.
6. Life is always a tragic story. Always the body slows, weakens, breaks. Always ends in death.
7. The dumb mantra sticks in my head: *Everyone dies alone.* But it isn't the dying that terrifies. It's living unseen, unloved, unpersoned.

8. And, too, an ignominious death creeps nightmarish under my skin. I will get old and older and oldest without dying. I will outlive everyone I know. Rattle dry in a hotplate apartment, pause on every stair to catch my breath. Nobody will notice I've died until the stink of my body sickens the hallway. I don't know why I care. I won't know anything anymore. No longer my problem.

9. This can happen even if I marry or partner again, even if it is a mature and ever-deepening union. One of us will die, and one of us will have to go on living.

10. Even my grandparents, together until the end, were sealed inside their separate suits of skin. There were infinite spaces between them.

11. It is impossible to keep yourself pristine, unchanged by the people you love. Most of us bend to love. This is only human and even generous. I don't know how to pinpoint the border between a humane shift, making space for another's needs, and an abdication of the self. A martyr's (wife's) sacrifice on the altar of love.

12. I may have too much rage, too much need, to live with someone on the sweet side of that border.

It is a horror to be alone, but loneliness is at the center of being human. When I was a kid, I realized that all of us are locked forever inside our own heads. I cried because I would never be able to sit behind another person's eyes, never fully enter another's consciousness. How terribly alone we are. And then I tried to forget it. I tried to fit myself into a man's imagination so completely that the borders between us would disappear—we would feel and think in concert like twins in the womb.

When I was married, I lay in bed next to my husband while he slept. I cried silently, held myself as still as possible so I wouldn't shake the bed. In the morning he would roll over, put his arm around me.

I didn't understand how I could feel so abandoned. I should have never been lonely again.

Now I sleep with my arms wrapped around a pillow. A pillow doesn't toss in bed. It won't cling to me, or snore. I make a conscious effort to take up the entire bed, and when I wake I stretch my arms and legs to all four corners.

Mom suffocated her rage until it nailed her to the bed. I let mine pull me forward, carrying my bed on my back. I might land myself in an emptiness as great as my mother's. An open question. Solitude is terror, and I am walking directly into its eye. But look. The picture I once held in my head, of Mom in some other life, Mom striding along a foreign street—that's me. That's my story.

I dress myself like Judith in necklace and bracelets. On my right ring finger is a moonstone set in a thick silver band. A birthday gift to myself. It's as sharp as Mom's ring on my left hand, brass knuckles.

A friend suggests I am my own wife.

No, I say. I am nobody's wife, not even my own.

Call it an anti-wedding ring.

Still, my face remains Utah-open. A man will always see an invitation there when all I mean is my own pleasure.

Tonight I'll walk to the beach near my new Portuguese home. In the dark my face can soften into itself. I'll dip my feet in cold water and feel the sea pull me outward, and for now it will be enough.

~

ACKNOWLEDGMENTS

THIS BOOK HAS HAD SEVERAL midwives (of all genders). Elizabeth Bernstein and Katie Boyle helped shape my mess of words into something worth reading. Murray Weiss and Kim Lim brought it squalling into the world as a real book. Trusted readers and swellest friends Dawn Oberg, Alia Volz, Jeneva Burroughs Stone, and Joe Loya gave me insight and cheer when I needed it most. Joe refused to believe me when I told him I couldn't write memoir. In trying to prove him wrong, it seems I wrote a memoir. Karen Erlichman has held my stories and helped me make them meaningful for over fifteen years. Roxane Gay published the essay that would grow into the heart of this memoir, and Chiwan Choi published a fictional account of a piece of this story. *Wiving* would not exist without you lovely humans.

Thank you, believers, supporters, inspirers: Nayomi Munaweera for a writing desk in a coconut grove. Kyle Smith and Julius Leiman-Carbia for a rooftop garden. Anne Schukat for my first step on the road. Joy Hanford, Alfredo Pereira, and my siblings Hank and Amália for dinners while editing. Tom McGuane, who told me not to get bored with my own story. Miri Nakamura for forest and desert. Glen David Gold for conversations about memoir, and Ayelet Waldman for an early spark of interest in the story. Jamileh Jamison for treating me like a real writer before I knew I was.

Damion Searls for MacDowell (I didn't know these improbable things called residencies existed!). Crimsonites who made my writing habit possible while paying the rent. Anna Borroz for herself.

Special thanks to my literary families:

Five Monkeys, my first friends in San Francisco, who brought me Christmas during my Days of Blood: Madhuri Tangirala, MaryBeth Lorence, Jill James, and Daniel Heath.

I grew up as a writer and learned about literary community behind the scenes at Litquake. Thanks to Jane Ganahl and Jack Boulware for making something gorgeous, and thank you to all the committee members and volunteers I collided with there. Particular thanks are due to Nina Lesowitz and Liam Passmore for telling me I needed to own my identity as a writer. You were right.

Portuguese Artists Colony, of course. We made something mighty swell together: Tim Bauer, Daniel (again), Leslie Ingham, Roxane Beth Johnson, Alix Lambert, Peter Orner, Shanthi Sekaran, Maw Shein Win, Alice Wu, Cary Tennis, Jason Bryan, Lauren Traetto, Benjamin Wachs, Damion (again), and Kristin Fitzpatrick. Our guest readers, live writers, musicians, and our audiences most of all.

DISQUIET International Literary Program made me fall in love with Portugal and begin to believe in a writing life.

Squawlums, Leporines, and all the reading and storytelling series that gave me a stage and a mic.

At MacDowell Colony, fairyland for artists, I began to write the thing that I denied for years was a memoir. I was wrong. Thank you to everyone who makes that place what it is, including the artists who made my brain sizzle.

To everyone who gave me a home in my nomadic years: I send you all the love in my body. There will be more love for you in the next book!

To the cafés, bars, hotels, cupcake shops, tea shops, and restaurants that welcomed me and my laptop, papers, books; who know right away to bring me a *meia de leite* and leave me to my corner for hours, sometimes all day: thank you forever.

Thank you to the people I've loved in my various messy ways. The love stories in this book are, of necessity, incomplete, and most of what makes them beautiful occurs offstage. The love stories of all kinds that are not in these pages are no less important. You animate me every day.

Thanks to my family. These pages show how things looked from my spot as the littlest Myer; you knew whole other universes. But the love among us is real, and the Myer humor has warped me in the best way. To my sister: you were my stand-in mom, and then you became my steadfast friend. So much love to you.

ABOUT THE AUTHOR

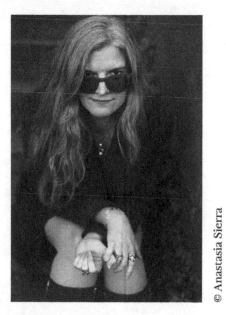

© Anastasia Sierra

CAITLIN MYER IS THE DAUGHTER of a poet and a visual artist, and she grew up in a large, chaotic Mormon family in Provo, Utah. Her short stories, poetry, and essays have appeared in *No Tokens*, *Electric Literature*, *The Butter*, *Cultural Weekly*, and *Joyland*, among others, and she was a 2012 MacDowell Colony Fellow. In 2010, Myer founded the San Francisco–based literary reading series, Portuguese Artists Colony (PAC), which has extended its reach beyond the US to performances in Portugal. For seven years she traveled the world, and she has recently settled in Guimarães, Portugal.